Renewal

A Story of Survival and Self-Discovery

Chris Moses

Renewal – A Story of Survival and Self-Discovery
© 2024 Chris Moses

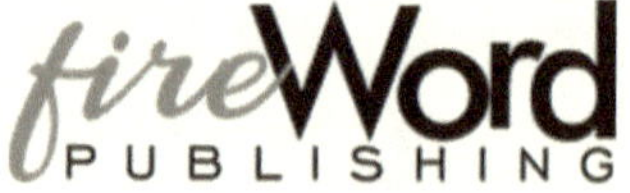

ISBN: 9798333145673

Acknowledgement

I would like to extend my heartfelt gratitude to Amanda Laughtland, my former professor and supervisor at Between The Lines Magazine, Edmonds Community College. Amanda's unwavering belief in my abilities and potential was instrumental in shaping my writing journey. Her nomination of me as Bilingual Literary Editor was a pivotal moment in my career and I am forever grateful for her trust and mentorship. Amanda's guidance, encouragement and support have had a lasting impact on my life and I am honored to acknowledge her influence on this book.

Thank you Amanda for being an exceptional educator, mentor and inspiration.

Table of Contents

Abstract

This memoir chronicles the transformative journey of a young athlete who, after a severe car accident, is forced to reevaluate his life. Raised under the contrasting influences of a supportive mother and a demanding father, he excels in soccer, earning a scholarship and the promise of a bright future. However, the pressures of competitive sports and neglect of personal well-being culminated in a life-altering accident and a shocking medical diagnosis. With the compassionate support of Mia, a nurse who later became his wife, Chris embarks on a path of self-discovery and healing. This story exemplifies the resilience of the human spirit, the power of love, and the significance of self-care and mindfulness.

Summary

Renewal is an inspiring story that takes readers through the life-altering experiences of the author. After surviving a severe accident and receiving a cancer diagnosis, the author embarks on a path of self-discovery and transformation, ultimately finding a deeper sense of purpose and fulfillment.

The story begins with the author stuck in a career chosen by his father, feeling unfulfilled and disconnected from his true aspirations. A sudden accident changes everything, leading to a hospital stay where he is diagnosed with cancer. This double blow forces him to reevaluate his life and search for deeper meaning.

In the hospital, the author discovers five key principles that help him through his darkest times. I have coined an acronym for these principles, which is GRACE. These principles became his foundation for recovery and personal growth.

- **G**lass Light.
- **R**ebirth from the Ashes.
- **A**bundant Connections: Nurturing Health Through Family and Gratitude.
- **C**oin Stand.

- **E**mpowering Autonomy: Embracing Your Desires to Navigate Life's Path.

After overcoming cancer, the author discovers his true calling: teaching others how to live healthier lives and prevent illnesses. He starts sharing his story and the GRACE principles with people worldwide, finding joy in helping others transform their lives.

The book ends with a powerful message to readers: embrace your true self, live with purpose, and apply the GRACE principles to overcome your own challenges. Through his journey, the author aims to inspire readers to pursue self-discovery, build resilience, and connect more deeply with their well-being.

Introduction

Life has a peculiar way of guiding us toward our true purpose, often through the most unexpected and challenging circumstances. This book is a testament to that journey—a story of transformation, resilience, and the profound realization that our greatest adversities can become the catalysts for our deepest self-discovery.

My name is Chris Moses, and this is my story. It begins not in a moment of triumph but in a period of profound despair. An accident, which I initially viewed as a disastrous setback, became the turning point that led me down a path of self-discovery and ultimately saved my life. Through this journey, I rediscovered my purpose and emerged with the mission to help others live a healthier and more fulfilling life.

It was an ordinary day, one of many I had spent pursuing a career that my father had envisioned for me. A career that, while prestigious and secure, had never truly resonated with my inner self. I had always felt an inexplicable void, a sense of unfulfillment that I couldn't quite articulate. But societal expectations and the desire to make my father proud kept me on this predetermined path.

In a split second, everything changed. I found myself in a hospital bed, grappling not only with physical injuries but also with a diagnosis that shook me to my core: cancer. The news slammed into me like a freight train, sending me spiraling into a deep void of fear and uncertainty. But it was in this abyss that I began to see the flicker of a new path. One that would lead me to a place of healing and profound self-discovery.

As I lay in that hospital bed, I was forced to confront my own mortality. It was a sobering experience. One that stripped away all the superficial layers of my life and brought me face-to-face with my true self. In the midst of this struggle, I stumbled upon a set of principles that would become my guiding light—principles I later encapsulated in the acronym GRACE.

As I emerged from my battle with cancer, I was not the same person who had entered that hospital. The experience had stripped away the illusions and brought me face-to-face with my true purpose. I realized that my calling was not the career my father had envisioned for me but something much deeper and more fulfilling:

teaching others how to live healthier lives and prevent illnesses.

This realization led me to a path of advocacy and education. I began sharing my story and the principles of GRACE with audiences around the world. I found immense joy and fulfillment in helping others discover their own paths to health and well-being. The very principles that had saved my life were now empowering others to transform theirs.

One of the most significant lessons I have learned on this journey is the importance of living authentically. For too long, I had lived according to the expectations of others, suppressing my true desires and aspirations. The accident and my subsequent battle with cancer forced me to confront this reality and embrace my authentic self.

Living authentically means being true to who you are, unapologetically. It means pursuing your passions, even when they defy societal expectations. It means valuing your own happiness and well-being above all else. This book is a call to action for anyone who feels trapped by the expectations of others or disconnected from their true self.

As you read my story, I invite you to embark on your own journey of self-discovery. Reflect on the principles of GRACE and how they can apply to your life.

Your journey may not involve an accident or a battle with cancer, but each of us faces challenges that can become opportunities for transformation. By embracing these principles, you too can discover your true purpose and live a healthier and more fulfilling life.

This is not just a book; it is a guide to transformation. It is a testament to the power of the human spirit and a roadmap for anyone seeking to rediscover themselves and live authentically. Through my story, I hope to inspire you to take control of your life, embrace your true self, and live with purpose and passion. **Welcome to the journey of rediscovering GRACE.**

PART ONE

Chapter 1: The Wake-Up Call

My life was forever changed on that fateful night of April 20, 2015, when I got into a rollover car accident en route to the HealthPoint Clinic in Bothell Washinton State. I was on a mission to retrieve my medical records, which were crucial for a job opportunity that promised to be rewarding. But what seemed like a minor obstacle at the time ended up being a turning point that would alter the course of my life forever. To truely understand the significance of that moment, one must first understand my background and the events that led me to that fateful night.

Growing up, my mom was my rock, my confidante and my guiding light. She was always there for me, supporting me through thick and thin, encouraging me to pursue my passions, and loving me unconditionally. In contrast, my dad was a different story. He was a former athlete himself and had high expectations for me to excel in sports from a young age. He pushed me hard to become a champion, just like him, using tough love and sometimes questionable methods. There were times when I felt like I was living his dream, not mine, but ultimately, his guidance helped me grow and develop as a person.

I thrived as an athlete despite the pressure. My natural talent was evident, and my mom's unwavering support gave me the confidence I needed to succeed. I tried my hand at multiple sports, but soccer quickly became my passion. I loved the rush of adrenaline that came with playing, the thrill of competing against other teams, and the sense of camaraderie that came with being part of a team. Soccer became more than just a sport for me; it was a way of life.

In my high school years, I was a shining star on the soccer field, and my exceptional skills caught the attention of several colleges who showed interest in recruiting me. My dad was overjoyed and beamed with pride, but my mom reminded me to remain humble, focus on my studies, and prioritize my happiness and personal growth as a young individual. Although I listened to the advice of my parents and coaches, the appeal of sports stardom was overwhelming. I knew that I had to chase my dreams, and my dedication paid off with a scholarship to a top university in Washington state. As a starting player on the soccer team, I gave it my all and left everything on the field.

In those glorious days, I felt invincible and on the verge of conquering the world. My future looked radiant, and nothing seemed impossible. However, as I became increasingly engrossed in the world of competitive sports, I gradually lost my sense of self and what truly mattered to me. The pressure to perform, the constant scrutiny, and the injuries during games took a toll on my mental and physical health. I started to neglect my relationships and my own well-being.

I was constantly on the pitch, pushing myself to the limit, but I didn't take breaks. I thought I was invincible, that I could handle anything that came my way. And my eating habits were far from healthy. I would grab fast food between practices, skip meals when I was too busy, and load up on energy drinks to keep me going. I thought I was fueling my body for success, but I was only damaging it in the long run.

And then, the accident happened. My world came crumbling down around me, and I forced to confront the destruction I had inflicted upon myself. The pain and suffering were overwhelming and I struggled to come to terms with the consequences of my actions.

I was exhausted from lack of sleep, distracted by my thoughts and recklessly speeding on that fateful day, trying to make up for lost time. The next thing I knew, I woke up in a hospital bed, surrounded by beeping machines and sterile white walls. The pain was excruciating, and my mind was foggy. I had no idea how long I had been out or what had happened.

As I gradually regained consciousness, I was told that I had broken my leg bone and had been in a coma for a period of three weeks. Following this, I received the distressing news that I had cancer cells in my liver, which would necessitate substantial changes to my lifestyle to fight the illness.

The diagnosis of a chronic illness served as a wake-up call, prompting me to recognize that I am not invincible. As I lay in that hospital bed, I realized that I had been living someone else's dream, not my own.

Amid adversity, Mia emerged as a beacon of hope, a compassionate nurse who attended to my injuries and offered a listening ear to my concerns. Her kind demeanor and soothing voice became my source of comfort during those trying times.

One day, as Mia was changing my dressing, I caught her gaze. I was struck by the kindness in her eyes and the softness of her features. In that moment, I felt a spark of attraction, but quickly looked away, unsure of how to process my emotions.

Mia noticed. She saw the flicker of admiration in my eyes and she looked away. She continued her work, trying to compose herself, but couldn't help sneaking glances at me.

Days passed, and my health began to improve. I started physical therapy and Mia was always there, encouraging me to push through the pain. One afternoon, as I was struggling to stand with my walker, Mia rushed to my side, supporting me with a gentle embrace.

I looked into her eyes, and this time, I didn't look away. Mia saw the love and gratitude in my gaze. Without a word, I wrapped my arms around her, holding her close as tears of joy and relief streamed down my face.

Mia's heart melted. She knew in that moment that she was falling in love with her patient, this broken and brave athlete had captured her heart. And as we held each other, the machines beeping in the background, our love story began.

Mia entered my life as my nurse and eventually became my lovely wife and mother of my two kids. She saw beyond my broken body and helped me find my strength again. Through her care and support, I discovered GRACE and began my journey towards self-rediscovery and growth. She was more than just a caregiver; she was a beacon of hope and support.

Mia's kindness, empathy, and compassion helped me find my strength again. She encouraged me to take small steps toward recovery, celebrating every tiny victory with me as I progressed.

The road to recovery was long and arduous. I was bedridden for months, unable to do the things I loved. I felt like a shadow of my former self, struggling to come to terms with my new reality. But I discovered the importance of self-care, mindfulness, and healthy habits. I learned to listen to my body, to prioritize my well-being, and to find joy in the little things. I began to see the world with fresh eyes.

As I reflect on my story, I see a young man who was lost in the spotlight, chasing a dream while letting every other part to the course of fate. But I also saw a survivor, a fighter, and a learner. I see a person who's found a new path, a new purpose, and a new love.

I realized that my accident was a wake-up call, a chance to reevaluate my priorities and find a new path. I had been living on autopilot, neglecting my health and relationships. And I hope that my story can inspire you to do the same – to find your strength, your own voice, and your own way.

This experience became the catalyst for my self-discovery and growth. I began to write about my journey, hoping to share my insights one day with others who might be struggling. I wanted to inspire them to take control of their well-being, to find their strength, and to live life to the fullest.

And so, my story begins, a testament to the power of resilience, love, and the human spirit. I invite you to join me on this journey, as we explore the ups and downs of life, the importance of self-care, and the transformative power of love and relationships.

Chapter 2: Chain Currency

Have you ever felt like your body and mind are connected in a way that's hard to explain? Like when you're stressed out, your body aches, or when you're happy, you feel more energized? That's because our physical, emotional, and mental well-being are all linked together like a chain. And just like a chain, if one link is weak or broken, the entire chain can suffer.

I learned this the hard way after my accident and was diagnosed with liver cancer. I had been neglecting my physical and emotional health for years, thinking I was invincible. But my diagnosis was a wake-up call, forcing me to confront the reality of my choices.

As I sat in my healing bed, facing the harsh reality of liver cancer, I realized that my neglect of my physical health and emotional well-being had finally caught up with me. I had been spending my "health currency" recklessly, ignoring the warning signs and pushing my body to its limits.

Funny enough, I wasn't alone in this. Many of us are guilty of this same behavior, prioritizing short-term gains over long-term well-being.

I remember when I first started experiencing symptoms of burnout. I was exhausted, anxious, and struggling to sleep. I thought to myself it was just stress from work, but looking back, I realize it was a sign that my Chain Currency was out of balance.

Understanding The Concept of Chain Currency

The concept of Chain Currency is simple: our physical, emotional, and mental health are all connected. Every thought, feeling and action has a ripple effect, influencing our overall well-being.

The concept of Chain Currency is rooted in the idea that our physical, emotional, and mental health are not separate entities but interconnected aspects of our overall well-being. Every action, thought, and emotion has a ripple effect, influencing our physical health, emotional state and mental clarity.

Think of it like a bank account. When we make healthy choices, we deposit them into our Chain Currency account. But when we neglect our well-being, we withdraw from that account. And if we're not careful, we can end up in debt—physically, emotionally and mentally.

The term "Chain Currency" refers to the intricate web of connections between our physical activities, emotional state and overall well-being. Just as a chain is made up of interconnected links, our health and well-being are linked to our emotional and physical activities. Every thought, feeling, and action sends ripples throughout our being, impacting our overall quality of life.

For me, the concept of Chain Currency hit close to home. I had always been someone who pushed herself to the limit, ignoring my physical and emotional needs in the process. I thought I was unreachable, that my body could handle anything I threw at it, but I was so wrong.

Physical activities, like exercise or poor posture, can impact our emotional state and mental well-being. For instance, regular exercise can boost our mood and energy levels, while poor posture can lead to physical discomfort and mental fatigue. I used to neglect my physical health, prioritizing work over self-care. But once I started paying more attention regularly and prioritizing my physical well-being, I noticed a significant improvement in my mental clarity and emotional resilience.

Emotional activities, like mindfulness or stress, can impact our physical health and mental clarity. Chronic stress, for example, can lead to physical symptoms like headaches and digestive issues, while mindfulness practices can improve our mental focus and emotional resilience. I used to struggle with anxiety and stress, but once I started practicing mindfulness and meditation, I noticed a significant reduction in my symptoms.

Mental activities, like negative self-talk or positive affirmations, can impact our emotional state and physical health. Negative self-talk can lead to emotional distress and physical tension, while positive affirmations can boost our mood and energy levels. I used to be guilty of negative self-talk, but once I started practicing positive affirmations, I noticed a significant improvement in my emotional well-being.

The Links in the Chain

The Chain Currency concept is made up of various links, each representing a different aspect of our physical, emotional, and mental well-being. These links are interconnected, and every action, thought, and emotion has a ripple effect throughout the chain.
Some of the key links in the Chain Currency include:

- Physical health: our physical body and its various systems, such as the cardiovascular, respiratory, and digestive systems.

- Emotional well-being: our emotional state, including our thoughts, feelings, and emotions.
- Mental clarity: our mental focus, concentration, and cognitive function.
- Spiritual connection: our sense of purpose, meaning, and connection to something greater than ourselves.
- Environmental influences: our external environment, including our social connections, work-life balance, and physical surroundings.
- Self-care practices: our habits and routines, such as exercise, nutrition, and stress management.

Breaking the Chain of Negative Patterns

Neglecting one aspect of our Chain Currency can lead to a breakdown in the entire system. For instance, neglecting our physical health can lead to emotional distress and mental fatigue. Similarly, neglecting our emotional well-being can lead to physical symptoms like headaches and digestive issues.

To break the chain of negative patterns, we must identify the weak links in our Chain Currency and address them. This may involve:

- Developing healthy self-care practices, such as regular exercise and balanced nutrition.

- Cultivating emotional resilience through mindfulness and stress management techniques.
- Improving our mental clarity through practices like meditation and positive affirmations.
- Nurturing our spiritual connection through activities like journaling and spending time in nature.
- Building a supportive environment through social connections and a healthy work-life balance.

Managing Our Chain Currency

Just as we manage our financial currency to achieve financial stability and security, we must learn to manage our Chain Currency to achieve optimal physical, emotional, and mental well-being. This involves:

- Being mindful of our thoughts, emotions, and actions.
- Practicing self-awareness and self-compassion.
- Setting boundaries and prioritizing our well-being.
- Cultivating healthy habits and routines.
- Seeking support and guidance when needed.

By understanding and managing our Chain Currency, we can break free from negative patterns and cultivate a life of vitality, resilience, and purpose. Remember, every thought, feeling, and action has a ripple effect. Let's make conscious choices by depositing into our Chain Currency account rather than withdrawing from it. Our well-being in the long run depends on it.

Just like time, each of us is given an equal amount of Chain Currency. We all have 24 hours in a day, and we all have the same opportunity to invest in our physical, emotional, and mental well-being. The difference lies in how we choose to spend our Chain Currency. Some people may think that they have less Chain Currency than others, but the truth is that we all have the same amount. It's just that some people are more mindful of how they spend it, and others are more reckless with their investments.

Some people may choose to lavish their Chain Currency on fleeting pleasures, like excessive screen time or unhealthy habits. We spend hours scrolling through social media, comparing our lives to others, and feeling inadequate. Or, we might indulge in unhealthy foods and drinks, ignoring the warning signs of our bodies. These choices may bring temporary happiness, but they ultimately drain our Chain Currency, leaving us feeling empty and unfulfilled. We might feel like we're getting a quick fix, but in reality, we're depleting our resources and harming our overall well-being. We're sacrificing our long-term health and happiness for a momentary high, and that's a dangerous trade-off.

On the other hand, others may invest their Chain Currency wisely, nurturing their relationships, learning new skills and taking care of their physical bodies through meditation, exercise and hobbies. They might cultivate meaningful connections with others, building strong relationships that bring joy and support. And they might pursue their passions, finding purpose and fulfillment in their work and activities. By making these choices, they're investing in their long-term happiness and well-being, rather than just seeking a quick fix. They're building a strong foundation for their lives, one that will support them through the ups and downs.

The beauty of Chain Currency is that it's entirely up to us how we choose to spend it. We can't blame genetics, circumstances, or external factors for our choices. We are the masters of our own Chain Currency and every decision we make has a ripple effect on our overall well-being. When we choose to invest in our well-being, we create a chain reaction of positivity that impacts every aspect of our lives. We feel more energized, more confident and more fulfilled. We're more resilient in the face of challenges, and we're more open to new opportunities and experiences. We're better equipped to handle stress and adversity and we're more likely to achieve our goals.

So, let's make conscious choices to invest our Chain Currency in activities that nourish our minds, bodies, and spirits. Let's prioritize self-care, build meaningful connections, and pursue our passions. By doing so, we'll create a chain reaction of positivity that will impact every aspect of our lives. We'll feel more alive, more purposeful, and more connected to ourselves and others. And we'll realize that our Chain Currency is a precious resource, one that we should cherish and invest wisely in. We'll be more mindful of how we spend our time and energy, and we'll make choices that align with our values and goals. We'll be more intentional about building strong relationships, and we'll cultivate a sense of community and belonging. We'll be more open to new experiences and opportunities, knowing that they have the potential to bring us joy and fulfillment.

Our Chain Currency is a precious resource, and it's up to us how we choose to spend it. Let's make conscious choices to invest in our well-being, relationships, and passions.

- How do you currently spend your Chain Currency? Are there any areas where you feel like you're wasting your resources?
- What are some ways you've been using your Chain Currency to seek temporary happiness?

- How has this impacted your overall well-being?
- What are some ways you've been investing your Chain Currency in your well-being and relationships? What are some areas where you'd like to improve?
- What are some choices you've made recently that have had a positive impact on your Chain Currency? What are some choices you regret making?

When we choose to invest in our well-being, we create a chain reaction of positivity that impacts every aspect of our lives. We feel more energized, more confident and more fulfilled. We're more resilient in the face of challenges and we're more open to new opportunities and experiences.

- How have you seen the concept of Chain Currency play out in your own life? What are some ways you'd like to invest your Chain Currency in the future?

By investing our Chain Currency wisely, we'll also be better equipped to handle the challenges that life throws our way. We'll be more resilient in the face of adversity, and we'll be more likely to bounce back from setbacks.

- What are the challenges you're currently dealing with? How could you use your Chain

Currency to build resilience and overcome them?

- What are some ways you've been investing in your relationships recently? What are some areas where you'd like to improve?
- What are some passions or interests you've been neglecting recently? How could you use your Chain Currency to pursue them?
- How do you commit to investing your Chain Currency wisely moving forward? What are some steps you can take today to start making positive changes?

PART TWO: GRACE

As we've explored the concept of Chain Currency and investing in our lives, we've laid the foundation for a fulfilling journey. We've seen how our choices and actions can either build a life of purpose, joy and vitality or lead us down a path of regret, dissatisfaction and poor health. But what does it look like to put these principles into practice? How can we apply the idea of Chain Currency to our daily lives in a way that brings about lasting change, transformation, and optimal well-being?

In the next chapter, we'll begin to dive into GRACE—the five life principles that have transformed my life and enabled me to achieve a healthier, happier, and more fulfilling existence. These principles have been forged in the fire of experience, shaped by the ups and downs of life, and refined through years of practice and reflection. They are the distillation of my journey, the essence of what I've learned and lived, and the keys to unlocking a life of purpose, joy and vibrant health for anyone, irrespective of age and race.

GRACE is not just a word; it's a way of life. These pillars form the foundation of a life well lived, a life filled with meaning, connection, and fulfillment.

In the following chapters, we'll explore each pillar of GRACE in depth, sharing practical strategies, insights, and exercises to help you integrate these principles into your own life. Together, we'll embark on a journey of self-discovery, healing, and transformation, unlocking the full potential of our Chain Currency and creating a life that is rich in every way.

As someone who has faced the challenge of cancer and emerged victorious, I can attest to the power of these principles for overcoming adversity and achieving optimal wellness. I've seen firsthand how these principles can help us navigate life's obstacles, build resilience, and cultivate a deep sense of purpose and meaning.

Today, I'm proud to say that I've transformed my habits and taken control of my chain currency. I'm investing in my own well-being, and it's been the best decision I ever made. I'm living proof that it's never too late to change and that our habits can either be our greatest asset or our worst enemy.

Join me as we explore the first principle, one that has been instrumental in my own journey towards wholeness and well-being. From the depths of struggle to the heights of triumph, this principle has been a constant companion, guiding me towards a life that is truly alive, vibrant, and full of purpose. Let's discover how embracing this principle can lead us to a life of freedom, happiness, and fulfillment, even in the face of challenges and uncertainty. Let's learn how to invest in our Chain Currency through GRACE and reap the rewards of a life that is rich in every way.

Chapter 3: Glass Light

A Poem on *Glass Light*

In the depths of darkness, a spark takes flight.
A glimmer of hope, a beacon in sight
A light that shines from within, pure and bright
Illuminating the path, guiding through the night

Like glass, we're fragile, vulnerable, and weak.
But with each crack, our strength and resilience speak.
We refract and reflect the light that we receive.
And radiate it outward, for all to perceive.

Our imperfections, the cracks that we bear
Become the windows through which our light shares
The beauty of our soul, the love that we hold
Shining like glass, young and old

In the fire of life, we're tempered and tried.
But like glass, we emerge stronger and more refined.
Our light shines brighter with each passing day.
As we embrace our vulnerabilities, in every way

So let us celebrate the cracks that we wear.
They are the proof of the light that we share.
And let our Glass Light, shine like a beacon high
Guiding us forward to a brighter sky.
As I continued on my journey, I realized that the concept of Chain Currency was not just about managing our physical, emotional and mental well-being but also about cultivating a sense of purpose and meaning. It's easy to get caught up

in the hustle and bustle of daily life, but what happens when we slow down and examine our inner selves? What do we find?

For me, the answer was a sense of disconnection. Despite my outward success, I felt unfulfilled and empty inside. It was as if I were living in a state of darkness, unable to see the beauty and light that surrounded me. I had been so focused on achieving my goals and meeting the expectations of my dad that I had neglected my own needs and desires. I was like a vessel without a spark.

After the accident, I was forced to confront a new reality. I had to rely on others for even the simplest tasks, and my sense of independence was shattered. But as I lay in bed, feeling helpless and alone, I realized that I had a choice to make. I could let my circumstances define me, or I could find a way to rise above them. It wasn't easy, but I started small. One day, I was hungry and was home alone, so I decided to make myself something to eat. It was a struggle, but I managed to drag myself into the kitchen and start cooking. As I stood at the stove, stirring the pot, I felt a sense of accomplishment that I hadn't felt in months.

Just as I was finishing up, Mia walked into the kitchen. She was taken aback by the sight of me standing there, cooking away. "Wow, you're a natural!" she exclaimed.

Her words struck a chord deep within me. I had been living someone else's dream not my own. I had always been passionate about cooking. During my early childhood, I would stay in the kitchen for hours with my mom and grandma, and we would prepare the most delicious delicacies ever. From rhubarb pie to seaweed flavor blasts, delicious old Indian menus, and lots more, but I had never pursued it as a career. Instead, I had followed the path that others had expected of me.

When I looked at Mia, I saw a spark of recognition in her eyes. She saw something in me that I had forgotten—my Glass Light. It was the spark within me that ignited my passions, values and purpose.

From that day on, Mia and I started cooking together. We experimented with new recipes and I discovered a sense of joy and fulfillment that I had never known before. Cooking became one of my therapies and my passion at this point.

And as we cooked, our relationship blossomed. Mia became not just my wife but also my partner in every sense of the word.

The accident was a blessing in disguise. It forced me to confront my inner self and discover my true passions. And it led me to Mia, who helped me see my Glass Light.

Glass Light represents the clarity and illumination that come from within. It's the spark that ignites when we align our actions and intentions with our deepest values and desires. It's the light that shines through the cracks of our brokenness, revealing our true strength and resilience. It's the radiance that emerges when we embrace our vulnerabilities and imperfections and allow ourselves to be seen and heard for who we really are or who we really want to be.

"As we venture deeper into the realm of self-discovery, we begin to uncover the hidden treasures of our inner world. The concept of Glass Light represents the delicate yet resilient nature of our inner selves, illuminating the path to our highest potential. Like a masterpiece of glasswork, our true essence is crafted with precision and care, reflecting the beauty and complexity of our human experience."

Just as glass can be fragile and vulnerable yet also strong and resilient, so too can we. When we embrace our vulnerabilities and imperfections, we open ourselves up to the possibility of transformation, growth and true joy. We become like glass, capable of refracting, and reflecting light in ways that illuminate our path and guide us forward. We become more aware of our thoughts, feelings and actions, and more intentional about the choices we make. We begin to see the world in a new light, as a place of wonder and possibility rather than a place of fear and limitation.

As I cultivated my own Glass Light, I began to notice changes in my life. I felt more confident, self-assured, and connected to myself and others. I was more creative and innovative, being at peace and joy with myself and more able to trust in the universe and its plan for me.

As we explore the concept of Glass Light, we'll delve deeper into the ways it can transform our lives.

Glass Light and the Art of Self-Reflection

As I cultivated my Glass Light, I realized that self-reflection was a crucial part of the process. I needed to take the time to examine my thoughts, feelings and actions, and to understand how they were impacting my life. I started journaling, meditating, and engaging in other practices that helped me tune into my inner world.

Through self-reflection, I discovered that I had been living someone else's dream rather than my own. I had been chasing success and validation from others, especially my dad, rather than listening to my own inner voice. I had been trying to fit into a mold that wasn't mine rather than embrace my unique shape and size.

As I let go of these external expectations and began to align with my own desires and values, my Glass Light began to shine brighter. I felt more confident, more authentic, and more at peace. I started to see the world in a new light, as a place of possibility and wonder rather than a place of fear and limitation.

Glass Light and the Power of Vulnerability

Vulnerability is a key component of Glass Light. I had to be willing to be vulnerable, to take risks, and to be seen and heard. I had to be willing to share my story, to reveal my imperfections, and to be authentic.

Through vulnerability, I discovered that I was not alone. I was connected to others, and we were all on this journey together. I felt a sense of community and belonging, and my Glass Light shone brighter as a result.

Glass Light and the Gift of Inner Wisdom

As I cultivated my Glass Light, I began to trust my inner wisdom. I started to listen to my intuition, to trust my instincts, and to follow my heart. I realized that I had the power to guide myself, to make decisions that were right for me, and to create the life I wanted. Through inner wisdom, I discovered that I was capable of so much more than I had ever imagined. I was strong, resilient, and powerful, and my Glass Light shone brighter as a result.

"Uncover the hidden treasures of your inner world and discover the radiant power of your Glass Light. Just like a delicate glass vase, our inner selves are often hidden from view, waiting to be discovered and cherished. But what happens when we finally uncover our Glass Light?"

My childhood friend Sarah, a thriving marketing executive who appeared to have everything in order, was struggling internally despite her outward appearance of confidence and self-assurance. Lacking direction and passion in her life, she felt like she was just going through the motions of her daily routine without purpose.

One day, Sarah called me and said, "I have decided to take a leap of faith and pursue my long-forgotten dream of becoming a writer." It was a scary and uncertain path, but she knew it was the only way to uncover her true potential, joy, and peace in nature. As she started writing, she felt a sense of joy and fulfillment that she had never experienced before. Her words were like a ray of light, shining bright and illuminating her path forward. Sarah's Glass Light was finally shining through, and it was radiant! She realized that her true purpose was not in marketing but in storytelling.

Sarah's story is relatable to many people, including perhaps you, the person reading this now, due to the train being crowded. Why not take the light and shine it on your delicate soul. As we uncover our own Glass Light, we may discover hidden talents, passions, and purposes that we never knew we had. We may find that our true calling is not what we expected, but that's what we need to truly be happy. And when we embrace our Glass Light, we become the radiant, confident, and purposeful individuals we were meant to be.

There's Always a Touch-Down Point

In my journey, I realized that my path to self-discovery was paved with the shards of a shattered dream. My dad, a one-time champ, had always painted a picture of all-time fame and glory, convincing me that sports were my ticket to success. And I bought into it hook, line and sinker I was so caught up in the thrill of competition, the rush of adrenaline, and the roar of the crowd that I forgot what truly brought me joy—cooking.

But I'm not alone in this struggle. So many of us are living a people-pleaser life, tilting away from our true nature and becoming mere mirages of ourselves. We're chasing the approval and validation of others, trying to fit into molds that weren't made for us. We're living someone else's dream, not our own.

My mom, wise and gentle, would often whisper words of wisdom in my ear. "Find joy and peace in whatever path you choose, son. Don't let others define your happiness." But I was only hearing her. I wasn't really listening to the message in her words. I was too busy chasing the spotlight, too consumed by the validation of others.

But life has a way of humbling us, doesn't it? Injury forced me to step away from the game, and I was left with nothing but time to confront the emptiness within. This was when I discovered the concept of Glass Light. It spoke to me on a deep level, resonating with my own experiences.

Glass Light represents the fragility of our desires and sense of purpose. Just like delicate glass, we can easily be swayed from our true passions and joys by the opinions and expectations of others if we don't constantly shine the light on our inner selves. We can become so focused on chasing the approval and validation of others that we lose sight of what truly brings us joy and fulfillment.

I know this all too well. I was so focused on living up to my dad's legacy on making him proud that

I forgot what truly makes me happy. And it wasn't until I let go of the need for external validation that I discovered my true passion for cooking.

But here's the thing: our Glass Light is not just a metaphor. It's a real and tangible light force within us. It's the spark that ignites our passions, values, and purpose. And when we nurture and trust our Glass Light, we begin to live a more authentic, meaningful, and fulfilling life.

My mom was right all along. Joy and peace are not found in external validation but in living a life true to ourselves. And it's never too late to discover our Glass, to embrace our true passions and desires.

In fact, it's often in the darkest moments, when our world is shattered like broken glass, that we are forced to confront our true selves. And it's in these moments that we have a choice: to pick up the pieces and try to glue them back together, or to use the shards to create something new, something beautiful, something true to who we are.

So many of us are living a life that's not truly ours, a life that's been shaped by the opinions and expectations of others. But it's never too late to break free from the mold and embrace our true selves. It's never too late to discover our Glass Light and live a life that's authentic, meaningful, and fulfilling.

Chapter 4: Rebirth from the Ashes

At this crossroads of my life, faced with the daunting diagnosis of cancer, I realized that I had two choices: succumb to the darkness or rise like a phoenix from the ashes. In this moment, I made vows to myself to transform my life, to leave behind the habits and beliefs that had held me back, and to embrace a new path to wellness and happiness.

In this chapter, I invite you to join me on a journey of rebirth and renewal as I share the powerful tools and strategies that helped me overcome the darkness and emerge stronger, wiser, and more radiant than ever before. From the depths of my struggles, I discovered a newfound appreciation for the simple yet profound practices of nutrition, movement, and mindfulness. These practices became my lifeline, guiding me back to wholeness and empowering me to live a life that is truly mine.

We'll explore the profound impact of movement on our physical, mental, and emotional well-being. We'll delve into the science behind exercise, revealing how it rewires our brains, strengthens our bodies, and nourishes our spirits. Through personal anecdotes, inspiring stories, and practical exercises, we'll guide you on a journey to discover the transformative power of movement.

Join me on this movement journey and discover the incredible power of exercise to transform your life. Let's rise from the ashes of our challenges and unleash our full potential, one movement at a time!

Through my story, I hope to inspire you to embrace your own transformation, to rise from the ashes of your challenges, and to unlock the power within you to create a life of purpose, joy, and fulfillment."

- *What is your current relationship with movement and exercise? Do you enjoy it, tolerate it, or avoid it?*

- *How has your body changed over the years? Have you experienced any significant physical transformations or challenges?*

- *What emotions or thoughts arise when you think about moving your body? Do you feel anxious, excited, or something else?*

- *Can you recall a moment when movement or exercise made you feel empowered, confident, or alive? What did that feel like?*

- *How do you think incorporating more movement into your daily routine could impact your mental and emotional well-being?*

- *What small step can you take today to initiate a transformation in your relationship with movement and exercise?*

Exercise is more than just physical activity; it's a potent tool that rewires our brains, boosting neuroplasticity and unlocking new pathways for growth. When we move our bodies, we stimulate our minds, releasing endorphins that elevate our mood, sharpen our focus, and enhance our creativity. By incorporating movement into our daily routine, we can improve cognitive function and memory, reduce stress and anxiety, increase self-esteem and confidence, and enhance our overall mental well-being.

As someone who once struggled with a sedentary lifestyle for a while, I know firsthand the transformative power of movement. When I started exercising regularly, I experienced a profound shift in my energy levels, my mood, and my overall sense of purpose. Movement became my sanctuary, and my confidence was boosted.

For many of us, the idea of transitioning from a sedentary lifestyle to an active one can seem daunting. We may feel stuck in our ways, unsure of where to start, or intimidated by the thought of exercising. But the truth is, making the transition to a more movement-filled life is not only possible, but it's also a crucial step towards achieving optimal wellness and happiness.

About ten months after the accident, as at this time I was at my second round of chemotherapy and I had also dropped one of my crushes. One faithful afternoon, when I came back from the hospital on an appointment with the doctor, I decided to take a small step towards reclaiming my physical health. I started practicing yoga, modifying the poses to accommodate my still-healing leg. It was tough at first, but gradually, I began to feel more flexible and stronger. Yoga was definitely a mind-and body-molding exercise for me because, with it, I was in touch with an inner me, and at the same time, I was stretching and taking baby moves again.

As I progressed in my yoga practice, I started thinking about other activities that brought me joy. *It was definitely cooking, of course.* I was already cooking for myself, and I realized that I could still pursue my passion for food even if I couldn't go back to sports due to the accident. So, I started taking cooking classes online and experimenting with new recipes.

Before long, I started a small catering business from my kitchen just to keep myself on the move, and soon, people were raving about my dishes. I had found a new sense of purpose and fulfillment in the kitchen, and I was grateful for the opportunity to share my creations with others while at the same time being on the move.

As I sat in my chair, staring at my computer screen, I couldn't help but think of my close friend, Alex. We had been friends since our early days, and I had seen him go through many ups and downs. But nothing could have prepared me for the transformation I witnessed in him over the past year.

Alex, a 40-year-old graphic designer, had spent most of his day sitting at a computer and his free time playing video games. As a result, he felt sluggish, tired, and struggled with back pain from sitting for long periods. One day, his wife encouraged him to join her for a hike on the weekends, which he bluntly refused. While on lunch with me a couple of days later, he said, "Buddy, my wife has been on my neck to go hiking with her, and I don't want to go." I asked him why he didn't want to go and he goes "Hmm... I don't know, but I don't feel like it. Maybe I would be too drained and tired when we return," all this he was saying while looking at the ceiling. I laughed and told him to give it a try and, afterward, give me feedback on how tired he was after the hike. He eventually agreed. A week later, when I called him to ask how it went, he was laughing and said to me, "I enjoyed the hike and felt invigorated afterwards."

This sparked a desire to incorporate more movement into his daily routine. Alex started small, taking short breaks every hour to stretch and move around. He also began doing push-ups and squats during commercial breaks while watching TV. Gradually, he increased his physical activity, joining a recreational soccer team and eventually training for a marathon.

I witnessed firsthand the significant improvements in his physical and mental health. He had more energy, his back pain decreased, and he felt more confident. He also lost weight and improved his overall well-being. I saw the spark in his eye return, and I knew that he was finding a new sense of purpose and fulfillment in his life.

Alex also made changes to his daily habits; he started taking walking meetings with clients instead of sitting in a conference room, using a standing desk at work and cycling to work instead of driving. These small changes added up to make a big impact on his overall health and wellbeing.

As I watched Alex's journey, I realized that sometimes all it takes is a small push to make a significant change. And for Alex, that push was his wife's encouragement to go for a hike. Now, he's a husband, father of three, and marathon runner—a true inspiration to me and everyone around him.

Alex's story illustrates how making small, incremental changes to your daily routine can add up to make a big impact on your overall health and wellbeing. By starting small and finding activities he enjoyed, Alex was able to sustain his new habits and make the transition to a more movement-filled life.

The Vision of Movement

Just like a runner visualizes crossing the finish line or a dancer envisions a flawless performance, we all have visions and goals that inspire us. These visions can be anything from starting a new business to improving our relationships or pursuing a passion project. They represent the destination we want to reach and the dream we strive to turn into reality.

However, having a vision alone is not enough; we must take movement steps to bring that vision to life. This is where the idea of movement comes into play. Movement in our everyday lives means making intentional choices and decisions that align with our goals. It's about taking that first step, no matter how small, towards creating the life we envision.

Just as physical inertia can make it challenging to get moving, mental and emotional inertia can hold us back from taking action in our lives. We may face resistance, self-doubt, or fear of failure.

But just like a body in motion tends to stay in motion, taking that initial step can break the inertia and set us on a path of momentum and progress.

Once we start moving towards our goals, be they body-shape goals, health goals, or even career goals, we begin to build momentum. Each action we take, no matter how small, adds to this momentum and propels us forward. It's like pushing a snowball down a hill - it starts small but gains speed and size as it rolls along. Similarly, our efforts compound over time, leading to significant progress and growth.

Embracing Consistency and Persistence

Consistency and persistence are key components of movement in everyday life. This also applies to our health. It's not just about making a single effort towards our goals but also about maintaining a steady pace and staying committed even when faced with challenges. By showing up consistently and persisting in our efforts, we create a rhythm of movement that keeps us moving towards success.

As we continue on our journey of movement towards our goals, it's important to celebrate milestones and acknowledge our progress. Whether it's reaching a specific target, overcoming a hurdle, or learning a new skill, each achievement fuels our motivation and reinforces our belief in our ability to succeed.

Ultimately, movement in everyday life is about adopting a mindset of continuous growth and improvement. It's about being proactive, taking initiative, and making the move to create the life and health we desire. By embracing movement as a way of life, we not only achieve our goals but also experience fulfillment, purpose, and a sense of accomplishment along the way.

So, what actions can you take today to create movement in your everyday life towards your vision and goals? It could be setting specific objectives, creating an action plan, breaking tasks into manageable steps, seeking support or mentorship, or simply taking that first courageous leap. Remember, every movement counts, and each step you take brings you closer to realizing your dreams. Let's harness the power of movement in our everyday lives and unleash our full potential!

It's essential to emphasize that movement encompasses far more than just physical exercise for a healthier body. It extends to every aspect of our lives, shaping our actions, decisions, and overall well-being. Movement is the force that propels us forward in pursuit of our visions and goals, driving us towards success and fulfillment.

Holistic movement encompasses not only physical activity but also mental, emotional, and spiritual growth. It's about making progress in all areas of our lives, from our careers and relationships to our personal development and self-care practices. When we embrace holistic movement, we align our actions with our values and aspirations, leading to a more balanced and fulfilling life.

Cultivating Mindful Movement

Mindful movement involves being present and intentional in our actions. It's about making conscious choices that support our well-being and contribute to our overall happiness. Whether it's practicing mindfulness meditation, engaging in meaningful conversations, or pursuing creative hobbies, every mindful movement we make adds richness and depth to our lives.

Life is filled with challenges and obstacles, but resilient movement allows us to navigate them with strength and determination. It's about bouncing back from setbacks, adapting to change, and learning and growing from adversity. When we approach life with resilient movement, we develop the inner fortitude and courage to overcome obstacles and thrive in the face of adversity.

Fostering Collaborative Movement

No person is an island, and collaborative movement involves working together with others to achieve common goals. It's about building meaningful connections, supporting one another, and creating positive change in our communities and society. When we foster collaborative movements, we harness the collective power of teamwork and cooperation to make a lasting impact on the world around us.

Celebrating the Journey of Movement

Lastly, it's crucial to celebrate the journey of movement itself. Each step we take, each milestone we reach, and each lesson we learn along the way contribute to our growth and evolution as individuals. Whether we achieve our ultimate goals or encounter detours and challenges, the journey of movement is what shapes us and defines our experiences.

In conclusion, movement is not just about physical exercise for a healthier body; it's a holistic approach to living a purposeful, fulfilling, and meaningful life. By embracing movement in every aspect of our lives, cultivating mindfulness, resilience, collaboration, and celebrating our journey, we unlock our full potential and create a life of joy, abundance, and fulfillment. Let's continue to harness the power of movement and make each moment count on our journey of growth and transformation.

Still Movement: Embracing

Rest as Vital to Rebirth

In the journey of rebirth from the ashes, one crucial aspect often overlooked is the importance of rest. While movement is essential for growth and transformation, so is the art of stillness and rejuvenation. Balancing the concepts of movement and rest is key to unlocking our full potential and experiencing true vitality.

Just as our bodies require physical movement to stay healthy and vibrant, they also need adequate rest to repair, recharge, and regenerate. Balancing movement and rest is like finding harmony in a symphony, where each note contributes to the overall composition of well-being.

The Rebirth Within Stillness

During periods of rest, our bodies are far from idle. They are engaged in a process of still movement, quietly but diligently working to replenish and renew. Cells regenerate, energy stores are replenished, and the mind finds clarity and peace. It's in these moments of stillness that the magic of rebirth truly takes place.

Quality rest is not just about sleeping; it's about giving ourselves permission to pause, unwind, and disconnect from the constant demands of life. In these moments, our bodies enter a state of deep relaxation, allowing for the restoration of energy and vigor. We wake up refreshed, revitalized, and ready to take on new challenges. It's the rebirth within stillness.

Rest is not merely a break from activity; it's an essential part of our journey to radiance. When we prioritize rest, our bodies have the opportunity to heal, rejuvenate, and glow from within. This radiance is not just skin-deep; it emanates from a place of balance and well-being that transcends outward appearance of glow and beauty.

The Dance of Movement and Rest

The dance of movement and rest is a continuous cycle, each complementing and enhancing the other. Just as movement propels us forward, rest anchors us in the present moment, allowing us to fully absorb and integrate our experiences. It's a dynamic interplay that keeps us in tune with our bodies, minds and spirits.

In embracing still movement, we honor the importance of rest as an integral part of our rebirth journey. It's not about constant activity or relentless pursuit; it's about finding the rhythm that works for us and allowing ourselves the grace to pause, reflect, and rejuvenate. In these moments of stillness, we discover new depths of resilience, clarity and inner strength.

Rest is not the absence of movement; it's a different kind of movement—a movement inward, a movement of restoration, and a movement of transformation. As we embrace the concept of still movement, we embrace the full spectrum of our humanity—the ebb and flow, the highs and lows, and the beauty of rebirth from the ashes.

Practical movement Exercises to Ignite Your Transformation

Ready to spark your transformation? Here are some practical movement exercises to get you started:

- *Morning Movement Rituals: Begin your day with a 10-minute movement routine, such as yoga, stretching, or a brisk walk.*
- *Find Your Flow: Engage in physical activities that bring you joy, whether it's dancing, swimming, or hiking.*
- *Move with Mindfulness: Combine movement with mindfulness techniques, such as meditation or deep breathing, to amplify the benefits.*

Chapter 5: Abundant Connections – Nurturing Health Through Family and Gratitude

In our pursuit of a healthier and happier life, we often focus on physical wellness, nutrition, and exercise. While these are essential components, there is another critical aspect that sometimes gets overlooked: our relationships. Building and nurturing strong, healthy relationships with our loved ones, family and friends can profoundly impact our well-being. This chapter, "Abundant Connection," explores the vital role of relationships and gratitude in achieving a balanced, joyful and fulfilling life.

When I reflect on my journey, I realize that the love and support of my family played an indispensable role in my healing and growth. After my cancer diagnosis, my family rallied around me, providing the strength and encouragement I needed to face the challenges ahead. This experience underscored for me how vital strong, supportive relationships are to our overall health and well-being.

Our relationships shape our experiences and influence our mental and emotional states. Positive relationships can provide a sense of security, belonging and purpose, while strained or negative relationships can lead to stress, anxiety, and even physical health issues.

Consider the story of the Johnson family, which serves as a poignant example of the impact of relationships on health and happiness. John and Lisa Johnson had been married for over a decade.

However, their relationship was far from harmonious. They frequently argued, and there was a persistent undercurrent of dissatisfaction and unhappiness. Both John and Lisa often expressed feelings of not being happy.

Years of unresolved conflicts and a lack of effective communication took a toll on their health. John, in particular, started experiencing symptoms of high blood pressure. The stress from their turbulent relationship was literally making him sick.

One day, I happened to observe the Johnsons from a distance. Their interactions were filled with tension and frustration. It was clear that their unhappiness was affecting not just their relationship but also their individual well-being. I saw in them a reflection of what happens when we neglect the importance of nurturing our connections with loved ones.

Realizing the need for change, John and Lisa decided to seek help. They attended couples therapy and learned how to communicate more effectively. They began to express gratitude for each other, focusing on the positive aspects of their relationship rather than dwelling on the negatives. Slowly but surely, their relationship began to improve. They started spending quality time together, rediscovering the love and affection that had brought them together in the first place.

As their relationship healed, so did John's health. His blood pressure stabilized, and he felt more at peace. Lisa also felt happier and more fulfilled. This transformation in their relationship highlighted the profound connection between emotional well-being and physical health.

Gratitude: The Glue That Binds

One Sunday afternoon, I was driving back home from church with Mia and our kids, Alexa and Dan. The car was filled with the joyous sounds of a gratitude song playing on the stereo. The kids were singing along enthusiastically, but it was Alexa who captured my attention. She was completely lost in the music, her little voice rising above the rest, her arms waving in the air as she sang along with pure, unfiltered joy. I glanced at the rearview mirror, watching her and feeling a deep sense of contentment.

At that moment, I felt a wave of gratitude wash over me. I was grateful for so many things: my loving and supportive wife, Mia, who had stood by me through thick and thin; my beautiful children, whose laughter and innocence brought light into our home; the opportunity to fight back against cancer and reclaim my health; not everybody is given that golden opportunity; and the thriving restaurant business that allowed me to pursue my passion for cooking. I was also thankful for the small moments, like the one I was experiencing right then, which reminded me of the beauty and joy in everyday life.

These reflections made me realize how crucial it is to acknowledge and cherish the seemingly insignificant things that make our lives meaningful. It's easy to get caught up in the challenges and setbacks we face, but finding gratitude in the little moments can help us stay grounded and focused on what truly matters.

One of the most powerful tools for strengthening relationships is gratitude. When we express appreciation for our loved ones, we reinforce positive feelings and foster a deeper connection. Gratitude helps us focus on the good in our relationships, promoting a more positive and supportive environment.

In my own life, I found that practicing gratitude transformed my relationships. When I started acknowledging the small acts of kindness from my family and friends, it not only made me feel more connected to them but also encouraged them to continue their supportive behavior. Gratitude creates a virtuous cycle of positivity that can significantly enhance our relationships.

Building Abundant Connections

Building and maintaining strong relationships requires effort, but the rewards are immense.

Here are some practical steps to cultivate abundant connections in your life:

1. Communicate Openly and Honestly: Effective communication is the cornerstone of any healthy relationship. Make an effort to listen actively and express your thoughts and feelings openly.

2. Spend Quality Time Together: Dedicate time to be with your loved ones without distractions. Engage in activities that you all enjoy and create lasting memories together.

3. Express Gratitude Regularly: Make it a habit to express appreciation for the people in your life. A simple "thank you" can go a long way in strengthening your bonds.

4. Support Each Other: Be there for your loved ones in times of need. Offering support and understanding can deepen your connection and build trust.

5. Resolve Conflicts Constructively: Disagreements are natural, but how we handle them makes a difference. Approach conflicts with a mindset of finding a resolution rather than winning an argument.

The concept of abundant connection is about recognizing and nurturing the relationships that enrich our lives. It's about creating a network of support, love, and gratitude that sustains us through life's challenges and joys. By fostering healthy relationships and expressing gratitude, we can create a foundation for a healthier, happier, and more fulfilling life.

As we reflect on the importance of relationships, let's commit to investing time and effort into building abundant connections. Let's appreciate the people in our lives, communicate openly, and support each other. In doing so, we not only enhance our well-being but also contribute to a more loving and connected world.

Abundant connection is at the heart of a healthy life. Our relationships provide the emotional sustenance we need to thrive. By focusing on building strong, positive connections and expressing gratitude, we can enhance our well-being and create a life filled with love, joy and fulfillment.

Reflecting on the Johnson family and my own experiences, I am reminded of the profound impact that relationships have on our health and happiness. Let's cherish and nurture our connections, embracing the abundant love and support that surrounds us.

Let's make a commitment to cultivate abundant connections in our lives. Let's appreciate our loved ones, communicate openly, and support each other through thick and thin. In doing so, we not only improve our own health and happiness but also contribute to the well-being of those around us.

The Heartbeat of Family: Everyday Moments of Abundance

Picture a typical day in your family's life. It could be the cheerful chaos of breakfast time, the warmth of a shared meal, or the comfort of a bedtime story. These moments may seem ordinary, but they are the threads that weave the tapestry of abundant connections within your family.

For me, it's the laughter that fills our kitchen during Sunday brunches with Mia and the kids, the heartfelt conversations during evening walks with my loved ones, or the joy of seeing my children grow and thrive. These simple yet precious moments remind me of the abundance of love, joy, and gratitude that family brings into our lives.

Gratitude isn't just a practice; it's a way of life. It's about noticing the small things. I remember a time when a friend reached out with a handwritten note of thanks, expressing gratitude for a small favor I had done. That simple act of appreciation filled my heart with warmth and reminded me of the power of gratitude in our relationships. It's these little moments that make life truly abundant and meaningful.

Within our families, gratitude plays a significant role in strengthening bonds and fostering deeper connections. It's about saying "I love you" not just in words but through actions, showing appreciation for the efforts and sacrifices made by our loved ones, and being present in moments of joy and sorrow.

Letting Go of Hurts: The Path to Genuine Gratitude and Happiness

In the journey towards wholeness, one of the most challenging yet crucial steps is letting go of past hurts. It's a process that requires courage and determination, but it is essential for fostering genuine gratitude and happiness. When we hold onto pain and resentment, it weighs us down, preventing us from fully experiencing the joy and contentment that life has to offer. Conversely, when we let go of these hurts, we make room for positive emotions that can lead to profound healing and overall well-being.

Holding on to past grievances can be a significant barrier to happiness. It keeps us anchored in negative experiences, making it difficult to appreciate the present and embrace the future. However, letting go is not about forgetting or minimizing the impact of these experiences. It's about acknowledging the pain, processing it, and choosing to move forward without letting it control our lives.

Scientific research has shown that chronic stress and negative emotions can have detrimental effects on our physical health. They can weaken the immune system, increase inflammation, and contribute to various chronic diseases. On the other hand, positive emotions such as happiness, gratitude, and love have been linked to numerous health benefits, including improved cardiovascular health, stronger immunity, and better overall longevity.

When we let go of emotional baggage, we create space for positive emotions to flourish. This shift can lead to the rebirth of healthy cells as the body responds to a more positive internal environment. Happiness and gratitude release endorphins and other feel-good chemicals in the brain, which promote healing and regeneration at a cellular level.

Letting go of hurt requires courage. It involves confronting your fears and being willing to face the pain head-on. This process can be difficult, but it is necessary for true healing and growth. By letting go, you are not only freeing yourself from the burden of the past but also paving the way for a brighter, more fulfilling future.

Practical Action Plan

Pause! *As you read this, I encourage you to take a moment to reflect on any past hurts or grievances that may be holding you back. Consider how letting go of these negative emotions could transform your life, allowing you to experience genuine gratitude and happiness. Remember, you have the power to choose your path and embrace the healing journey ahead.*

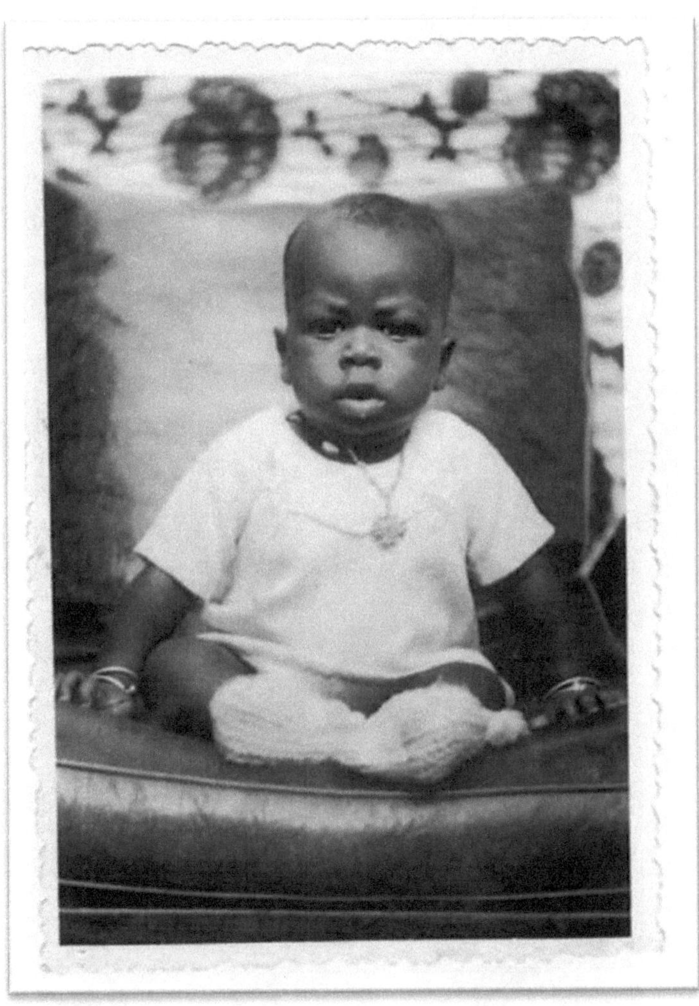

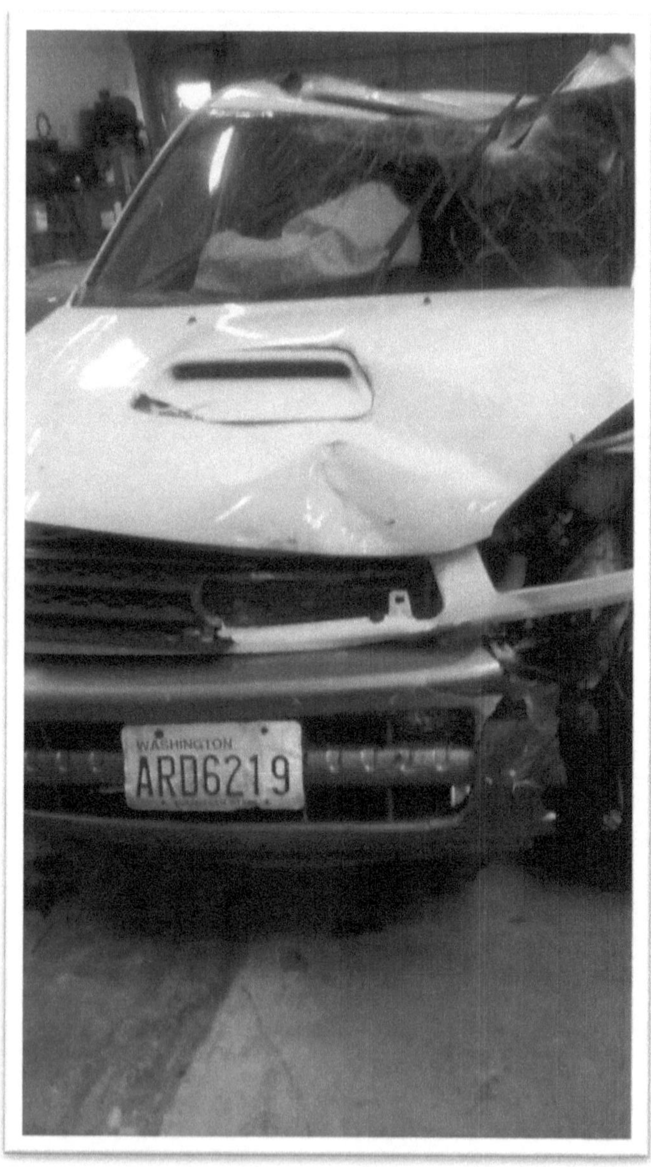

WASHINGTON
ARD6219

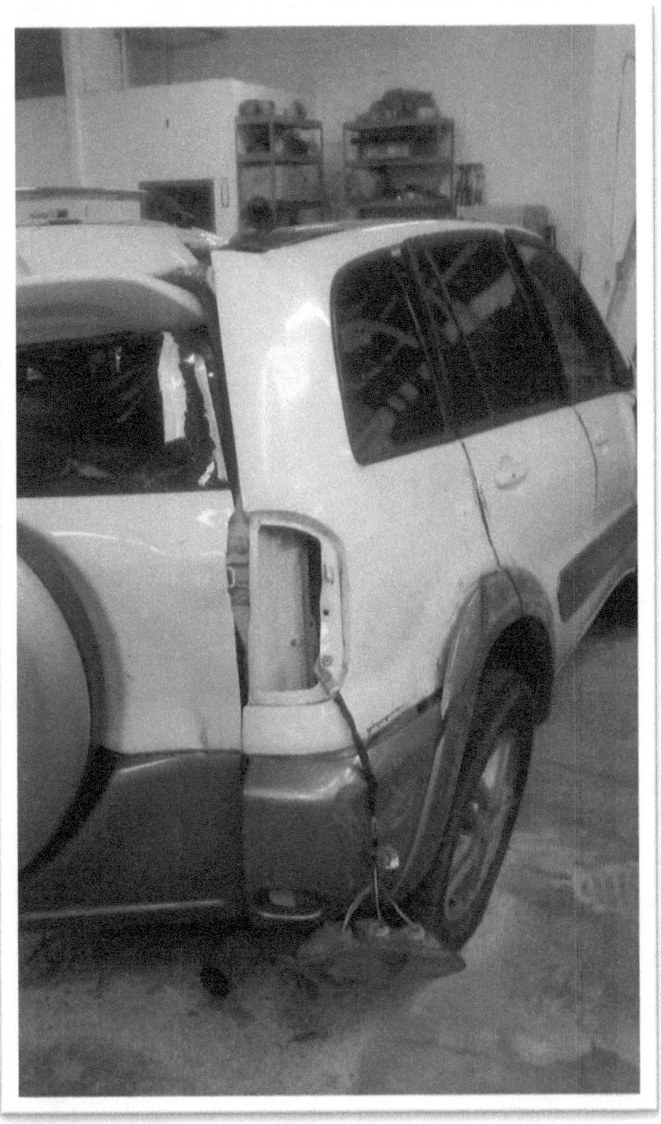

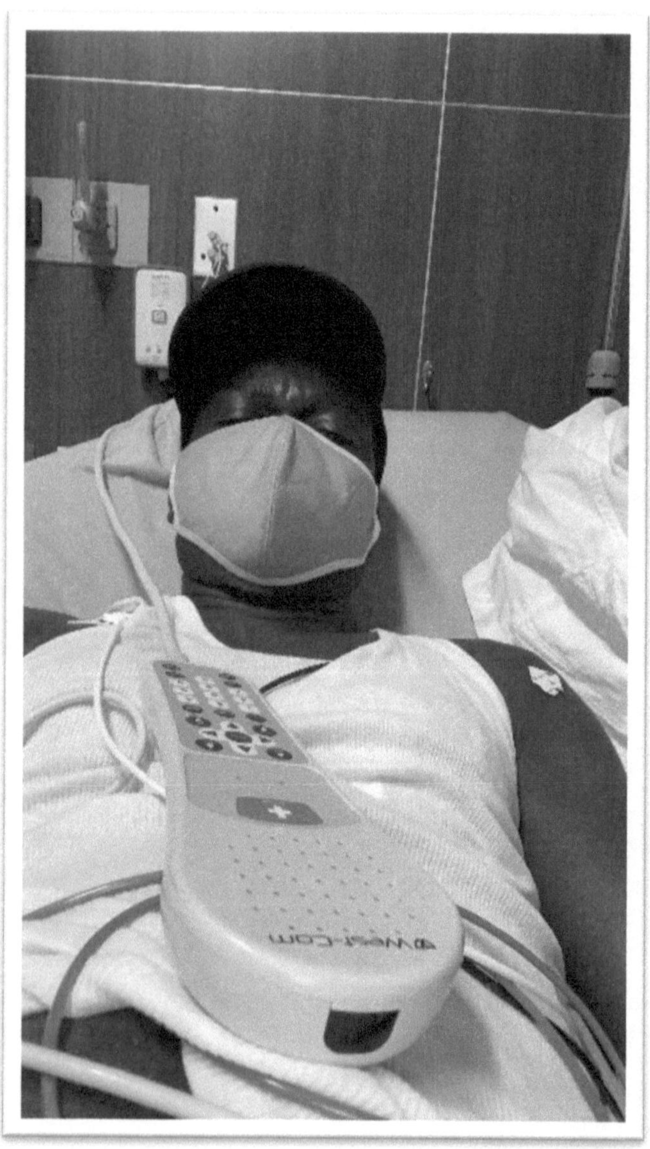

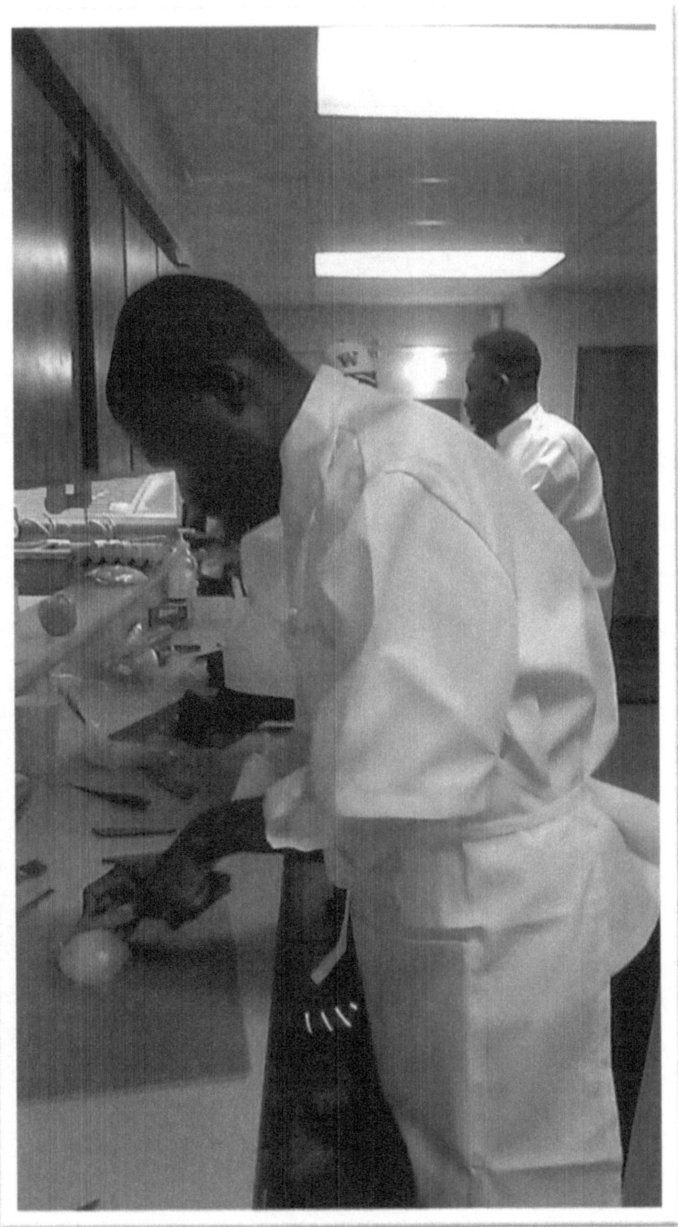

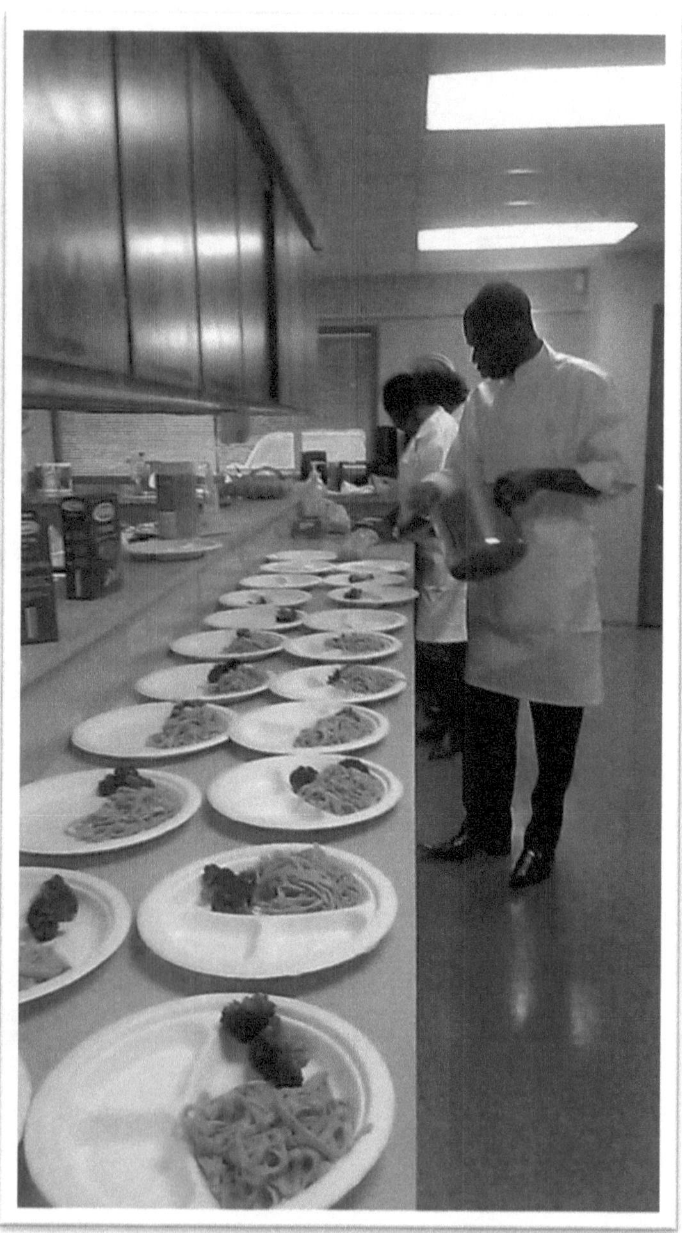

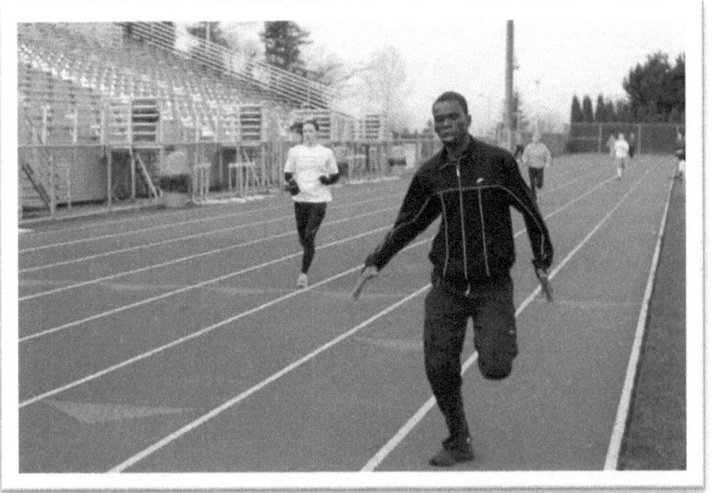

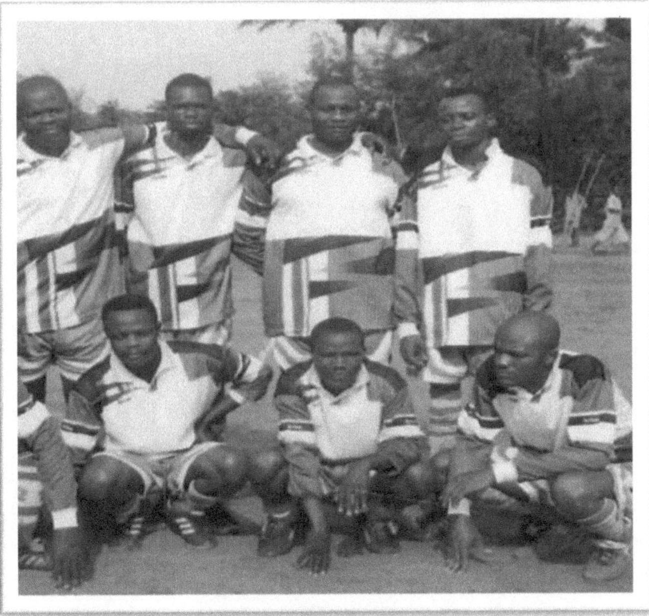

Chapter 6: Coin Stand

In this chapter, we explore the delicate art of balancing our everyday lives. Just like a coin standing on its edge, maintaining balance in life requires mindfulness and intentional effort. Whether it's managing work and personal life, finding the right mix between activity and rest, or nurturing relationships while taking care of oneself, balance is key to a fulfilling and healthy existence. Too much of anything—work, rest, stress, or even pleasure—can lead to imbalance and ultimately harm our well-being.

The Concept of Balance

Life is often likened to a coin, with two distinct sides representing the dualities we encounter. On one side, there's the hustle and bustle of everyday life—career ambitions, relationships, and personal goals. On the other hand, there's the need for rest, self-care, and inner peace. Striking a balance between these two sides, much like standing a coin on its edge, is a lifelong journey filled with challenges, lessons, and moments of profound insight.

Balance is essential for stability. Imagine trying to balance a coin on its edge. It requires patience, precision, and a delicate touch. Similarly, achieving balance in life involves careful consideration of various aspects, including physical health, mental well-being, relationships, work and leisure. It's about creating a harmonious existence where all parts are in sync, supporting and complementing each other.

The journey to finding balance begins with acknowledging the multifaceted nature of life. It's a quest that encompasses various aspects, each requiring attention and nurturing. From career aspirations to personal passions, relationships, health, and well-being, achieving equilibrium involves a delicate dance of priorities and choices.

Returning to work after triumphing over cancer marked a significant milestone in my life. It was a moment of empowerment and reflection, where the importance of self-care became paramount. Balancing professional commitments with personal well-being meant reevaluating priorities, setting boundaries, and fostering a supportive work environment.

Nurturing Relationships: Communication, Boundaries, and Growth

Post-cancer recovery reshaped my perspective on relationships. While the love and support were unwavering during challenging times, maintaining balance required clear communication and boundary-setting. Expressing needs, respecting personal space, and fostering mutual growth became pillars of healthy, fulfilling relationships.

The pursuit of holistic wellness became a cornerstone of my journey. It wasn't just about physical health but also nurturing mental and emotional well-being. Adopting a balanced diet, incorporating regular exercise, practicing mindfulness, and seeking professional support when needed contributed to overall vitality and resilience.

Embracing Change and Flexibility: Lessons from Life's Ebb and Flow

Life is dynamic, marked by constant change and adaptation. Embracing change meant letting go of old habits and beliefs that no longer served growth. It meant remaining flexible, open to new experiences, and resilient in the face of challenges.

Inner balance has become a daily practice rooted in self-awareness and self-care. Mindfulness practices, gratitude journaling, and moments of quiet reflection became anchors in the quest for inner harmony. Embracing vulnerability, practicing self-compassion, and honoring emotions contributed to a deeper sense of peace and authenticity.

Life's journey is a tapestry woven with contrasting threads: success and failure, happiness and sadness, love and loss. These dualities are what make our experiences rich and meaningful. Just as a coin has two sides, we encounter moments of light and shadow. The key is not to be consumed by either extreme but to find harmony in the middle ground.

Reflecting on my own life, I've experienced the highs of success and the lows of adversity. The exhilaration of overcoming challenges is balanced by the humbling lessons learned from failures. ***Each victory is tempered with gratitude, while every setback becomes a stepping stone for growth. It's this delicate dance between opposites that shapes our resilience and character.***

One of the most common areas where balance is crucial is maintaining good health while pursuing ambitious goals. In today's fast-paced world, it's easy to get caught up in the pursuit of success at the expense of well-being. I've learned firsthand that neglecting health for the sake of ambition is a precarious path.

As I was declared cancer-free five years after the accident and embarked on the journey of rebuilding my life, I faced the challenge of striking a balance between health and ambition. The intense focus on recovery often clashed with the drive to achieve new milestones in my career. It was a delicate tightrope walk, requiring mindful decisions and prioritization.

1. ***The Power of Prioritization:*** *Balancing life's demands necessitates prioritizing what truly matters. Just as I prioritized my health during recovery, it's vital to identify core values and allocate time and energy accordingly.*

2. ***The Myth of Perfection:*** *Striving for perfection in every aspect of life can lead to burnout and dissatisfaction. Embracing imperfection and accepting setbacks as part of the journey fosters resilience and self-compassion.*

3. ***Mindfulness in Action****: Practicing mindfulness cultivates awareness of the present moment, allowing for better decision-making and reduced stress. Incorporating mindfulness practices, such as meditation or deep breathing, can enhance overall well-being.*

4. ***Nurturing Relationships and Self-Care:*** *Another crucial aspect of balance is nurturing meaningful relationships while practicing self-care. Neglecting either can lead to feelings of loneliness or burnout. Building strong connections with loved ones provides support during challenging times, while self-care rituals replenish energy and foster inner peace.*

During my recovery phase, I leaned heavily on the support of family and friends. Their presence provided emotional nourishment and reminded me of the importance of nurturing relationships. Concurrently, prioritizing self-care activities like meditation and nature walks rejuvenated my spirit and maintained balance.

1. ***Boundaries and Self-Care:*** *Setting boundaries in relationships and honoring personal needs are integral to maintaining balance. It's okay to say no and prioritize self-care without guilt.*

2. ***Quality over Quantity:*** *cultivating a few deep, meaningful relationships is more fulfilling than spreading oneself thin across numerous connections. Dedicate your time and effort to what truly matters.*

3. ***The Ripple Effect:*** *Balancing personal well-being positively impacts relationships and vice versa. When we are grounded and content, our interactions with others reflect harmony and authenticity.*

Life is in constant flux, marked by moments of change and transformation. Embracing impermanence allows for flexibility and adaptation. What once seemed insurmountable may evolve into an opportunity for growth. The coin of life spins, revealing new facets with each turn.

The journey post-cancer brought significant changes, both internally and externally. Embracing the impermanence of circumstances allowed for a mindset shift from fear to curiosity. Each change, whether small or monumental, became a catalyst for personal growth and self-discovery.

1. ***Flexibility and Adaptability***: *resisting change only leads to frustration. Embracing the ebb and flow of life with flexibility opens doors to new experiences and insights.*

2. ***Learning from Challenges***: *Every challenge offers a lesson. Instead of perceiving setbacks as failures, see them as opportunities to learn and build resilience.*

3. ***Embracing Uncertainty:*** *Life's uncertainties can be unsettling yet liberating. They remind us of our resilience and capacity to navigate the unknown with courage and grace.*

The Dangers of Extremes: Finding Balance in a World of Extremes

In our modern world, the pervasive issue that plagues humanity is our tendency to veer towards extremes. We yearn for power, wealth, success, and validation, often going to extreme lengths to attain these desires. However, this relentless pursuit of extremes often leaves us depleted, disconnected, and disillusioned. It's a cycle of highs and lows, with little room for sustainable fulfillment and contentment.

One of the primary areas where we witness the dangers of extremes is in the pursuit of power. Whether it's political power, social influence, or authority in various spheres of life, the thirst for power can drive individuals and societies to extreme measures. We see this play out in the realms of politics, business, and even personal relationships, where the quest for dominance can overshadow empathy, collaboration, and ethical conduct.

Similarly, the relentless pursuit of wealth often leads to extremes of overwork, financial stress, and materialism. We sacrifice our well-being, relationships, and even our values in the pursuit of financial success. The allure of money blinds us to the true riches of life: meaningful connections, inner peace, and purposeful living.

In moments of anger or conflict, our emotions can drive us to extremes of hurtful words, aggression, or even violence. The inability to manage our emotions and communicate effectively leads to ruptured relationships, emotional scars, and deep-seated regrets. It's in these moments of heated passion that we lose sight of empathy, understanding, and constructive dialogue.

Another aspect of extremes manifests in our lifestyle choices. We oscillate between periods of neglecting our well-being, be it physical, mental, or emotional, and moments of overindulgence to compensate for the neglect. We starve ourselves of self-care, only to binge on unhealthy habits when the pressure mounts or when crisis strikes. This cycle perpetuates a sense of imbalance and dissatisfaction.

The Path to Balance: Early Intervention and Mindful Living

Breaking free from the grip of extremes requires a conscious effort to cultivate balance in every aspect of life. It begins with early intervention, recognizing the signs of imbalance before they escalate into crises. Rather than waiting until our health, relationships, or mental well-being deteriorate, we must prioritize preventive measures and holistic self-care.

Mindfulness emerges as a potent tool for navigating the complexities of modern life. By cultivating awareness of our thoughts, emotions, and actions, we gain insight into our patterns of behavior and can course-correct before veering off into extremes. Mindfulness prompts us to pause, reflect, and respond with thoughtfulness instead of reacting impulsively.

At the core of finding balance is embracing moderation and restraint. It's about finding the sweet spot between ambition and contentment, between productivity and rest, between passion and equanimity. Practicing moderation allows us to savor life's experiences without being consumed by excess or scarcity.

When we prioritize balance in our lives, we create a ripple effect of positivity that extends beyond ourselves. Balanced individuals contribute to harmonious relationships, ethical decision-making, and a more sustainable society. It's a collective journey towards equilibrium, where each individual's commitment to balance contributes to a healthier, happier world.

The essence of the "coin stand" analogy is captured in the concepts of early intervention and mindful living. Just as a coin stand requires steady attention to remain upright, our lives demand proactive measures to prevent extremes. Mindfulness serves as a stabilizing force, helping us stay centered amidst life's fluctuations and challenges.

So here is the thing: life's balance is not a static state but a dynamic dance of adaptation and mindfulness. By honoring dualities, nurturing relationships, practicing self-care, and embracing impermanence, we navigate the coin's edge with grace and wisdom. By recognizing the pitfalls of imbalance and embracing a lifestyle of moderation, mindfulness, and early intervention, we pave the way for a more harmonious existence. Just as a coin stands tall on its edge, so too can we find equilibrium amidst life's myriad experiences. Remember, like a coin standing on its edge, balance requires patience, mindfulness, and a gentle touch. The journey continues, each step a testament to resilience, growth, and the beauty of balance.

Chapter 7: Empowering Autonomy – Embracing Your Desires to Navigate Life's Path

In a world brimming with diverse perspectives and competing narratives, one of the most profound acts of self-empowerment is embracing your desires as the compass guiding your journey through life. The "E" in this chapter stands for Empowerment, highlighting the importance of taking ownership of your path, choices, and aspirations. Let's delve into the empowering journey of defining your own narrative and navigating life's complexities on your terms.

From a young age, we are often bombarded with external expectations and societal norms that shape our beliefs and choices. Family, peers, and society at large may have well-intentioned but sometimes limiting ideas about what constitutes success, happiness, or fulfillment. However, true empowerment begins when you recognize that your desires, dreams, and passions are valid and worthy of pursuit.

Imagine a scenario where societal norms dictate that success can only be achieved through a traditional career path. Despite having a passion for the arts, you may feel pressured to conform and pursue a more conventional route. However, embracing your desires means defying external expectations and charting a course aligned with your true calling, even if it diverges from the norm.

Empowerment stems from honoring your inner guidance and intuition. It's about tuning into your deepest desires, values, and convictions to make choices that resonate with your authentic self. This inner compass serves as a steadfast guide, steering you toward experiences, relationships, and endeavors that align with your purpose and vision for life.

Consider moments in your life when you've felt a deep sense of alignment and fulfillment. Perhaps it was pursuing a hobby that ignited your passion, forging genuine connections with like-minded individuals, or making a bold decision that honored your values. These moments of clarity and conviction are reflections of your inner guidance at work, guiding you toward a life of meaning and purpose.

Empowerment often involves embracing risk and cultivating resilience in the face of challenges. It means stepping outside your comfort zone, taking calculated risks, and learning from setbacks and failures. While the path of empowerment may not always be smooth or straightforward, each experience contributes to your growth, strength and resilience.

Think about a time when you took a leap of faith, pursued a new opportunity, or overcame a significant obstacle. These moments of courage and resilience are emblematic of your empowerment journey. By embracing risk and resilience, you expand your horizons, discover new capabilities, and forge a path uniquely your own.

Cultivating Self-Awareness and Authenticity

Empowerment thrives in the soil of self-awareness and authenticity. It's about knowing yourself—your strengths, weaknesses, values, and passions—and living in alignment with your true essence. Cultivating self-awareness involves introspection, reflection, and a willingness to explore your inner landscape without judgment or inhibition _*that is turning on your Glass Light.*

Authenticity, in turn, is the art of living congruently with your values, beliefs, and aspirations. It's about showing up as your genuine self, expressing your truth, and honoring your uniqueness. When you embody authenticity, you attract experiences and relationships that resonate with your authentic vibration, fostering deeper connections and fulfillment.

While empowerment entails honoring your desires and authenticity, it also involves navigating external influences with discernment. External factors such as societal norms, cultural expectations, and peer pressure may attempt to sway your decisions or define your worth. However, true empowerment lies in discerning which external influences align with your values and aspirations and which ones detract from your empowerment journey.

For instance, social media often presents curated narratives and unrealistic standards that can impact self-esteem and self-worth. Empowerment involves consuming media mindfully, discerning between genuine inspiration and detrimental comparison, and curating a digital environment that uplifts and empowers you.

Reflecting on my own empowerment journey, I recall pivotal moments when embracing my desires transformed my path and perspective. One such moment was deciding to pursue a passion project despite initial doubts and external skepticism. Embracing my desire to create and share my voice in writing led to a sense of fulfillment and purpose that transcended external validation.

Another empowering experience was learning to set boundaries and prioritize self-care. Embracing my desire for balance and well-being meant saying no to commitments that drained my energy and yes to activities that nourished my soul. This shift in mindset empowered me to reclaim my time, energy and autonomy.

Navigating external influences has been an ongoing aspect of my empowerment journey. By discerning which voices and narratives resonate with my truth and which ones detract from it, I've cultivated a digital and social environment that supports my growth and well-being. Empowerment, for me, is a dynamic and evolving journey of self-discovery, resilience and authenticity.

Empowerment is not a destination but a lifelong journey of self-discovery, growth, and authenticity. By embracing your desires as the guiding force in your life, you empower yourself to navigate challenges, cultivate resilience, and live authentically. Your empowerment journey is unique to you and shaped by your experiences, choices, and aspirations. Embrace it with courage, curiosity, and a commitment to honoring your true self.

Embracing Your Own Perspective: Resisting the Urge to Fit In

In the quest for empowerment and authenticity, one of the most liberating practices is resisting the urge to fit into other people's perspectives or expectations. This section delves into the importance of embracing your own perspective, accepting what you cannot change, and focusing your energy on meaningful transformations within your control.

The Futility of Fitting In

Throughout life, we encounter diverse perspectives, opinions, and expectations from those around us. Family, friends, colleagues, and society at large may have preconceived notions of how we should think, behave, or live our lives. However, the pursuit of fitting into these molds often leads to a sense of disconnection from our true selves; it results in a sense of emptiness or lack of fulfillment because it doesn't align with our authentic desires and values.

Empowerment begins when you embrace your uniqueness and resist the pressure to conform to external standards or norms. Each individual possesses a unique set of experiences, talents, passions, and perspectives that shape their identity and journey. Embracing your uniqueness involves celebrating your strengths, accepting your limitations, and owning your narrative without seeking validation or approval from others.

Quick action point

Pause! *Think about the qualities or aspects of yourself that make you unique. It could be your creativity, empathy, resilience, or unconventional approach to life. Embracing these qualities allows you to stand out authentically and contribute your unique gifts to the world, rather than striving to fit into a predetermined mold.*

Empowerment also involves accepting aspects of life or circumstances that are beyond your control. This includes external factors such as others' opinions, societal expectations, or past experiences that cannot be altered. While you cannot change these externalities, you can change your perspective and response and focus on what you can control. For example, if someone holds a negative opinion of you or misunderstands your intentions, you cannot control their perception or behavior. However, you can control how you choose to respond—with grace, understanding, and a focus on your own growth and well-being.

Focusing on Meaningful Change

Empowerment thrives when you redirect your energy toward meaningful changes within your control. This includes personal growth, self-improvement, pursuing passions, cultivating healthy relationships, and contributing positively to your community or causes you believe in. By focusing on meaningful change, you reclaim agency over your life and create a ripple effect of empowerment in your environment.

Quick Action Point

Pause! *Consider areas of your life where you can initiate meaningful change. It could be setting personal goals for growth, practicing self-care and self-compassion, fostering authentic connections with others, or advocating for causes that align with your values. These intentional actions fuel your empowerment journey and inspire others to embrace their uniqueness and agency.*

Reflecting on my own journey and embracing my perspective has been a transformative aspect of empowerment. I recall moments when I resisted the urge to conform to external expectations or seek constant validation.

One pivotal moment was realizing that I couldn't control how others perceived me or my food at the restaurant all the time. However, I could control the effort I put into my passions for cooking every single time I am given the beautiful opportunity to cook, the authenticity of my contributions, and the impact I aim to create.

Strategies for Embracing Your Own Perspective

1. **Self-Reflection:** Take time for introspection and self-reflection to understand your values, desires, and aspirations without external influence.

2. **Practice Self-Validation:** Cultivate self-compassion, self-acceptance, and self-validation to rely less on external validation for your worth or identity.

3. **Focus on Growth:** Redirect your energy toward meaningful growth, personal development, and contributions that align with your values and passions.

4. **Let Go of Control:** Accept aspects of life beyond your control, including others' opinions or circumstances, and focus on what you can influence positively.

5. **Surround Yourself Wisely:** Surround yourself with supportive, like-minded individuals who celebrate your uniqueness and empower your journey.

The 69 of Life: Diverse Perspectives

Imagine the number 6 or 9 written on a piece of paper. For some, it appears as a six, while for others, it's a nine. Neither perspective is wrong; they simply represent different angles of perception. Similarly, in life, our experiences, beliefs, and interpretations shape our unique viewpoint of the world. Understanding that others may see things differently—like a 69—helps foster empathy, respect, and open-mindedness.

Recently, I found myself in a situation that underscored the importance of viewing life from diverse perspectives. A neighbor had constructed a fence that encroached slightly on my property line. Initially, I felt a surge of anger and injustice, ready to confront the neighbor and demand immediate rectification.

However, before reacting impulsively, I paused to consider the situation from the neighbor's perspective. I realized that he might have constructed the fence unintentionally or without realizing the property boundaries. Taking a moment to empathize with his possible viewpoint shifted my approach from confrontation to communication.

Instead of launching into a heated argument, I chose to initiate a calm and respectful conversation with my neighbor. I expressed my concerns about the fence's placement and asked if we could find a mutually agreeable solution. This approach, rooted in empathy and understanding, transformed a potential conflict into a collaborative problem-solving endeavor.

During our discussion, I listened attentively to my neighbor's perspective. He shared his intentions behind the fence's placement and acknowledged the oversight regarding property boundaries. Together, we devised a plan to adjust the fence slightly to adhere to the correct property lines without escalating tensions or animosity. This experience taught me valuable lessons about embracing diverse perspectives and reframing conflicts through empathy.

1. **Empathy Fosters Understanding**: By empathizing with others' viewpoints, we gain a deeper understanding of their intentions, motivations and challenges.

2. **Communication Over Confrontation:** Choosing open and respectful communication over immediate confrontation fosters constructive dialogue and collaborative solutions.

3. **Finding Common Ground:** Viewing situations from diverse perspectives helps identify common ground and facilitates mutually beneficial resolutions.

Quick Action Point

Consider instances in your own life where you've felt pressured to conform to others' expectations or opinions. Perhaps it was choosing a career path, navigating relationships, or adhering to societal standards of success. Reflect on how embracing your unique perspective, like a 69, can lead to greater authenticity, fulfillment, and empowerment.

Embracing Your 69 Perspective: Strategies for Empowerment

1. **Self-Reflection:** Take time for introspection to understand your values, beliefs, and aspirations without external influence.

2. **Empathetic Listening:** Practice active listening and empathy to understand others' viewpoints and foster meaningful connections.

3. **Conflict Resolution:** Approach conflicts with an open mind, seeking understanding, common ground, and mutually agreeable solutions.

4. **Resisting External Pressures:** Refrain from succumbing to societal pressures or expectations that don't align with your authentic self.

5. **Celebrating Diversity:** Embrace the diversity of perspectives around you, recognizing that different viewpoints enrich our collective experience.

Your Unique Perspective, Your Empowerment!

In conclusion, empowerment blooms when you embrace your own perspective, resist the urge to fit into external molds, and focus on meaningful changes within your control. Your uniqueness is your power—celebrate it, honor it, and let it guide your path authentically. By embracing your perspective, accepting what you cannot change, and focusing on meaningful transformations, you cultivate a life of authenticity, agency, and empowerment that inspires others along the way. Embrace your 69 mindset, celebrate diversity, and let your unique perspective guide you towards a life of fulfillment, connection and empowerment.

PART THREE: GRACEFUL PLATE

Welcome to the Graceful Plate, where we delve into the transformative power of food and nutrition in nurturing a vibrant and fulfilling life. Food is not just sustenance for our bodies; it is a cornerstone of well-being, vitality, and radiant health. In this chapter, we will explore the principles of mindful eating, nourishing our bodies with wholesome foods, and cultivating a harmonious relationship with what we consume.

Imagine a plate filled with vibrant colors, textures, and flavors—a symphony of nourishment that not only delights the senses but also fuels our vitality. This is the essence of the Graceful Plate, where every meal is an opportunity to nourish not just our bodies but also our souls.

In today's world, it's easy to overlook the importance of mindful eating. We often find ourselves rushing through meals, grabbing convenience foods, and neglecting the profound impact that our food choices have on our health and well-being. But by embracing the Graceful Plate philosophy, we can transform our relationship with food and unlock its full potential to heal, energize, and rejuvenate us from within.

Join me on a journey of culinary exploration as we discover the art of mindful eating, the benefits of whole foods, and the simple yet powerful practices that can elevate our health, vitality, and glow. Let's savor each bite, nourish our bodies with intention, and celebrate the abundance of flavors and nutrients that nature provides.

In our quest for health and happiness, the role of food cannot be overstated. The adage "You are what you eat" is more relevant today than ever before. The Graceful Plate is not just about the food we eat but about choosing nourishing, healing foods that support our body's natural processes. It's about understanding that what we give to our body as food will come back to us in the form of energy, vitality, and overall well-being.

The Graceful Plate represents a holistic approach to eating that prioritizes nutrient-rich, whole foods. It's a way of eating that goes beyond merely filling our stomachs; it's about feeding our bodies with the nutrients they need to thrive. This concept emphasizes balance, variety, and mindfulness in our food choices, ensuring that each meal is a step towards better health and healing.

Before discovering the Graceful Plate, I was on a different path. My eating habits were influenced by convenience, cravings, and a lack of awareness about the profound impact of nutrition on health. It took a serious health challenge—my battle with cancer—to truly understand the importance of what I was feeding my body. The transformation that followed was nothing short of life-changing.

Whole foods are the foundation of the Graceful Plate. These are foods that are as close to their natural state as possible, free from excessive processing, artificial additives, and preservatives. Think fresh fruits and vegetables, whole grains, nuts, seeds, legumes and lean proteins. These foods are rich in essential nutrients, including vitamins, minerals, fiber, and antioxidants, which are crucial for maintaining health and supporting the body's healing processes.

During my recovery, I embraced whole foods wholeheartedly. I started my day with a colorful smoothie packed with leafy greens, berries, and a handful of nuts. Lunch often consisted of a hearty salad with a variety of vegetables, whole grains like quinoa, and a source of lean protein. Dinner was a balanced meal of steamed vegetables, grilled fish, and a portion of brown rice. This shift towards whole foods provided my body with the nutrients it needed to heal and regain strength.

Chapter 8: The Healing Power of Food

The Graceful Plate is particularly focused on the healing power of food. Certain foods have been shown to support the body's natural healing processes, reduce inflammation, and boost the immune system. For example, foods rich in antioxidants, such as berries, dark leafy greens, and nuts, can help protect the body from oxidative stress and cellular damage. Omega-3 fatty acids found in fish, flaxseeds, and walnuts are known to reduce inflammation and support heart health.

During my cancer treatment, I incorporated many healing foods into my diet. Turmeric, known for its powerful anti-inflammatory properties, became a staple in my meals. I added ginger to my teas and smoothies for its immune-boosting benefits. Leafy greens like spinach and kale provided essential vitamins and minerals, while berries offered a sweet, antioxidant-rich treat.

Grace Mindful Eating

Mindful eating is a key component of the Graceful Plate. It entails giving complete attention to the act of eating and drinking, focusing on both internal and external sensations. This means being entirely present during meals, relishing each mouthful, and tuning in to your body's signals of hunger and satiety. This practice can help prevent overeating, improve digestion, and enhance the overall enjoyment of food.

For me, mindful eating was a revelation. Instead of eating on the go or while distracted by screens, I began to set aside time for meals, focusing solely on the food and the company of loved ones. I learned to appreciate the flavors, textures, and aromas of each dish. This shift not only improved my digestion but also made meals a more enjoyable and fulfilling experience.

The Graceful Plate also emphasizes balance and moderation. While it's important to choose nutrient-dense foods, it's equally important to enjoy a variety of foods and not to deprive oneself. Deprivation can lead to cravings and unhealthy eating patterns. Instead, the Graceful Plate encourages a balanced approach, where all foods can fit into a healthy diet in moderation.

My journey with the Graceful Plate taught me the importance of balance. I learned to enjoy occasional treats without guilt, understanding that a healthy diet is about overall patterns rather than perfection. This balanced approach made it easier to sustain healthy eating habits in the long run.

My discovery of the Graceful Plate was a gradual process, born out of necessity and fueled by a desire for better health. The wake-up call came when I was diagnosed with cancer. The initial shock and fear were overwhelming, but they were soon replaced by a determination to fight back. I realized that, in addition to medical treatment, I needed to support my body through proper nutrition. This was the beginning of my journey with the Graceful Plate.

I started by educating myself about the role of nutrition in cancer treatment and recovery. I consulted with nutritionists, read books, and researched extensively. The more I learned, the more I understood that my diet needed a complete overhaul. I began to eliminate processed foods and introduce more whole, nutrient-dense foods into my meals.

One of the most significant changes was my breakfast routine. Instead of sugary cereals or pastries, I started my day with a smoothie packed with leafy greens, berries, chia seeds, and a scoop of plant-based protein powder. This nutrient-rich breakfast provided me with the energy and nutrients I needed to start the day strong.

Lunch and dinner became opportunities to experiment with new recipes and ingredients. I discovered the joy of cooking with fresh vegetables, herbs, and spices. I learned to prepare balanced meals that included a variety of food groups, ensuring that my body received a wide range of nutrients. I also made a conscious effort to include healing foods, such as turmeric, ginger, garlic, and green tea, known for their anti-inflammatory and antioxidant properties.

As I continued on this path, I noticed significant improvements in my health and well-being. My energy levels increased, my immune system strengthened, and I felt more resilient in the face of treatment. The Graceful Plate not only supported my recovery but also transformed my relationship with food. I began to see food as medicine, a powerful tool for healing and nourishment.

Tips for Embracing the Graceful Plate

1. **Prioritize Whole Foods:** Choose fresh, whole foods over processed and packaged options. Include a diverse array of fruits, vegetables, whole grains, lean proteins, and healthy fats in your diet.

2. **Cook at Home:** Preparing meals at home allows you to control the ingredients and cooking methods, ensuring that your food is nutritious and free from unnecessary additives.

3. **Practice Mindful Eating:** Take time to savor your meals, paying attention to the flavors, textures, and aromas. Listen to your body's hunger and fullness cues to avoid overeating.

4. **Stay Hydrated:** Drink plenty of water throughout the day to support digestion, circulation, and overall health. Avoid sugary beverages and limit alcohol consumption.

5. **Incorporate Healing Foods:** Include foods known for their healing properties, such as leafy greens, berries, turmeric, ginger, garlic, and green tea.

6. **Balance and Moderation:** Enjoy a variety of foods in moderation. Allow yourself occasional treats without guilt, focusing on overall patterns rather than perfection.

7. **Listen to Your Body**: Pay attention to how different foods make you feel. Each person's body is unique, so what suits one individual might not suit another. Tailor your diet to meet your specific needs and preferences.

In conclusion, the Graceful Plate is more than just a way of eating; it's a philosophy that embraces the power of food to heal, nourish, and rejuvenate. By prioritizing whole, nutrient-dense foods, practicing mindful eating, and maintaining balance and moderation, we can transform our health and well-being. My journey with the Graceful Plate taught me that what we give to our bodies as food, they will give back to us in the form of vitality, resilience, and overall health.

As you embark on your own journey with the Graceful Plate, remember that every meal is an opportunity to nourish your body and support your health. Embrace the abundance of flavors and nutrients that nature provides, and celebrate the joy of eating mindfully and intentionally. Here's to a vibrant, healthy, and graceful life, one plate at a time.

The Graceful Plate: Beyond Food Choices

While the concept of the Graceful Plate emphasizes the importance of nutritious, whole foods, it also highlights a significant truth: some people pay little attention to what they eat but are still keen to avoid weight gain or health challenges. They indulge in unhealthy eating habits and then feel compelled to spend hours at the gym to offset their dietary choices. This cycle of indulgence and guilt-driven exercise is not only unsustainable but also a form of self-deception.

Many individuals find themselves trapped in a pattern where they eat without mindfulness, often consuming foods high in sugar, unhealthy fats, and empty calories. These eating habits may provide temporary pleasure but ultimately lead to feelings of guilt and the need to compensate through intense exercise. Unfortunately, this approach can create a cycle of unhealthy behaviors that are hard to break.

I've seen this firsthand on my own journey. Before embracing the Graceful Plate, I often indulged in convenience foods and sugary treats, thinking I could simply "burn it off" later at the gym. However, this mindset led to a constant struggle with my weight and energy levels. No matter how much I exercised, I couldn't outwork a poor diet.

The reality is that our bodies need more than just calorie burning to stay healthy. Exercise is crucial, but it should be a tool for maintaining fitness, enhancing mental well-being, and improving overall health—not a punishment for dietary indulgence.

When we focus on eating well, we naturally reduce the need for extreme measures to maintain our weight and health. Consuming a balanced diet rich in whole foods provides our bodies with the essential nutrients they need to function optimally. This means we can enjoy the benefits of exercise without the pressure of compensating for poor eating habits.

Here's the transformative insight: *when you nourish your body properly, you won't need to* *spend hours at the gym to "burn off" what you've eaten. Instead, exercise becomes a positive, enjoyable part of your routine, aimed at keeping fit and enhancing your well-being, rather than a form of punishment.*

I learned this lesson the hard way. During my battle with cancer, I had to re-evaluate my approach to food and exercise. I realized that my body needed real, nutrient-rich food to heal and regain strength. Once I adopted the principles of the Graceful Plate, I found that my energy levels stabilized, my weight was easier to manage, and my workouts were more effective and enjoyable. The key to breaking the cycle of guilt-driven exercise is to change our relationship with food and fitness. Here are some strategies to help you make this shift:

1. **Adopt the Graceful Plate Philosophy**: Focus on incorporating whole, nutrient-dense foods into your diet. This will provide your body with the fuel it needs to thrive without the need for excessive exercise to offset poor food choices.

2. **Mindful Eating:** Pay attention to what you eat and how it makes you feel. Engage in mindful eating by enjoying each bite and paying attention to your body's hunger and fullness signals. This can prevent overeating and reduce the need for guilt-driven exercise.

3. **A Balanced Approach to Fitness:** Exercise should be a celebration of what your body can do, not a punishment for what you've eaten. Find physical activities you enjoy and incorporate them into your routine for the sheer pleasure and health benefits they provide.

4. **Set Realistic Goals:** Focus on setting achievable fitness goals that are not tied to compensating for dietary indulgences. Aim for overall health and wellness rather than specific weight-loss targets driven by guilt.

5. **Consistency Over Intensity:** Consistent, moderate exercise is more sustainable and beneficial in the long run than intense, sporadic workouts motivated by guilt. Find a routine that you can maintain without feeling overwhelmed or exhausted.

6. **Support System:** Surround yourself with supportive friends and family who understand your goals and can provide encouragement. Having a support system can help you maintain healthy habits more easily.

Allow me to share a personal experience that highlights this point. During my cancer recovery, I was determined to regain my strength and fitness. Initially, I pushed myself hard at the gym, thinking that intense workouts would speed up my recovery. However, I soon realized that this approach was actually counterproductive. My body was already under stress from treatment, and adding more stress through excessive exercise only made things worse.

I decided to shift my focus to the principles of the Graceful Plate. I began eating nutrient-rich foods that supported my healing process and adopted a more balanced approach to exercise. Instead of punishing my body with grueling workouts, I engaged in gentle activities like yoga, walking, and light strength training. This allowed my body to recover at its own pace and improved my overall well-being.

The results were remarkable. Not only did I feel stronger and more energetic, but I also developed a healthier relationship with food and exercise. I no longer felt the need to compensate for my dietary choices with intense workouts. Instead, I enjoyed the process of nourishing my body and staying active in ways that felt good and sustainable.

Here are some practical tips to help you embrace the Graceful Plate and achieve sustainable health:

1. **Plan Your Meals:** Take time to plan your meals and snacks, focusing on whole, nutrient-dense foods. This can help you avoid the temptation of convenience foods and ensure that

you're nourishing your body with the nutrients it needs.

2. **Enjoy the Process:** Find joy in the process of preparing and eating healthy meals. Experiment with new recipes, explore different cuisines, and make mealtime an enjoyable experience.

3. **Listen to Your Body:** Observe how your body reacts to various foods and activities. Since everyone is unique, it's essential to discover what works best for you.

4. **Practice Self-Compassion:** Be kind to yourself and recognize that it's okay to indulge occasionally. The key is to enjoy these moments without guilt and to return to your healthy habits without feeling like you've failed.

5. **Focus on Overall Wellness:** Remember that health is about more than just diet and exercise. Prioritize sleep, stress management, and mental well-being as part of your overall approach to health.

The Graceful Plate in Everyday Life

Incorporating the Graceful Plate into your everyday life doesn't have to be complicated. It's about implementing small, sustainable changes that accumulate over time. Here are some examples of how you can apply the principles of the Graceful Plate in your daily routine:

• **Breakfast:** Start your day with a nutrient-rich smoothie or a bowl of oatmeal topped with fresh fruit and nuts. This provides a balanced mix of carbohydrates, protein, and healthy fats to fuel your morning.

• **Lunch:** Prepare a colorful salad with a variety of vegetables, whole grains, and a source of lean protein. Add a drizzle of olive oil and a squeeze of lemon for a burst of flavor.

• **Dinner:** Enjoy a balanced meal that includes a variety of food groups. For example, you could have grilled salmon with roasted vegetables and a side of quinoa. This ensures that you're getting a range of nutrients to support your health.

• **Snacks:** Choose healthy snacks like fresh fruit, nuts, or yogurt. These options provide sustained energy and prevent the need for unhealthy, processed snacks.

• **Hydration:** Stay hydrated by drinking plenty of water throughout the day to support your body's natural processes. Adding herbal teas and infused water can provide variety and flavor.

Love Your Body and Health—Treat It with Respect to Glow

Our bodies are incredible, capable of so much, and deserving of our utmost respect and care. However, in the hustle and bustle of daily life, it's easy to neglect our health and take our bodies for granted. We push ourselves to the limit, ignore signs of distress, and often prioritize other commitments over our well-being. But to truly thrive and glow, we must shift our mindset and treat our bodies with the love and respect they deserve.

Self-love is a transformative force that can radically improve our lives. It involves recognizing our worth, honoring our needs, and making choices that promote our well-being. When we love ourselves, we naturally adopt healthier habits, make better food choices, and engage in activities that nurture our bodies and minds.

My own journey taught me the importance of self-love. During my battle with cancer, I realized that I had often neglected my health, prioritizing work and other responsibilities over my well-being. This realization was a turning point. I began to practice self-love by listening to my body, making mindful food choices, and engaging in activities that promoted healing and relaxation.

Respecting your body means acknowledging its needs and treating it with kindness and care. It involves understanding that your body is your most valuable asset and that taking care of it should be a top priority. Here are some ways to treat your body with respect:

1. **Listen to Your Body:** Pay attention to how your body feels and responds to different foods, activities, and environments. Listen to its signals and adjust your habits accordingly.

2. **Prioritize Sleep:** Quality sleep is essential for overall health and well-being. Make sure to get sufficient restful sleep each night to enable your body to recover and rejuvenate.

3. **Stay Hydrated:** Drinking plenty of water is crucial for maintaining bodily functions and overall health. Prioritize staying hydrated throughout the day.

4. **Move Regularly:** Engage in regular physical activity that you enjoy. Whether it's walking, dancing, yoga, or strength training, find ways to move your body and stay active.

5. **Practice Stress Management:** Stress can have a significant impact on your health. Incorporate stress-reducing practices such as meditation, deep breathing, and mindfulness into your routine.

6. **Nourish with Whole Foods:** Focus on eating a balanced diet rich in whole, nutrient-dense foods. Avoid processed foods, and make mindful choices that support your health.

Before I discovered the concept of graceful eating, I often ate on the go, barely paying attention to what or how much I was consuming. My meals were rushed, and I rarely took the time to enjoy them. This changed during my cancer recovery when I realized the importance of mindful eating for my healing process.

I began to approach mealtime with intention and mindfulness. I made it a point to sit down for my meals, savor each bite, and appreciate the nourishment my food provided. This shift not only improved my digestion and energy levels but also transformed my relationship with food. Eating became a source of joy and nourishment rather than a mere necessity.

Moreover, practicing graceful eating can help prevent overeating and promote a healthy weight. By paying attention to hunger and fullness cues, we can avoid the common pitfall of eating out of habit or emotion. This balanced approach to eating supports long-term health and helps us maintain a healthy relationship with food.

Overcoming Challenges to Graceful Eating
While the principles of graceful eating are simple, implementing them can be challenging, especially in our fast-paced, convenience-driven society. Here are some strategies to help you overcome common obstacles:

1. **Plan Ahead:** Take time to plan your meals and snacks in advance. This can help you make healthier choices and avoid the temptation of convenience foods.

2. **Set Realistic Goals:** Start with small, achievable goals, such as eating one mindful meal a day or incorporating more vegetables into your diet. Gradually develop these habits over time.

3. **Create a Supportive Environment:** Surround yourself with people who support your healthy eating goals. Share meals with family and friends who appreciate the importance of nutritious, mindful eating.

4. **Practice Patience:** Changing your eating habits takes time and effort. Be kind to yourself and understand that progress may take time. Celebrate small victories along the way.

5. **Seek Professional Guidance:** If you're struggling to make healthy changes, consider seeking guidance from a nutritionist or dietitian.

They can offer customized guidance and assistance to help you reach your objectives.

As you continue your journey with the Graceful Plate, remember that every meal is an opportunity to practice self-love and respect. Embrace the art of graceful eating, savor the nourishment your food provides, and celebrate the positive impact it has on your health and well-being. Here's to a life of vitality, joy, and grace—one mindful bite at a time.

Sample Meals for Cancer Recovery

Here are some sample meals designed to aid in the treatment and recovery of cancer patients over the course of a year. These meals are structured to provide balanced nutrition, support immune function, and promote overall well-being.

Months 1–3: Nutrient-Dense and Easy-to-Digest Meals

Breakfast: Oatmeal topped with fruit and nuts; scrambled eggs served with whole wheat toast.

Lunch: Grilled chicken or fish with quinoa and steamed vegetables; lentil soup with whole grain bread.

Dinner: Roasted vegetables with lean beef or turkey, brown rice, and green beans.

Snacks: Fresh fruits, nuts, and carrot sticks with hummus.

These meals focus on providing lean proteins, whole grains, and a variety of colorful vegetables. The inclusion of easy-to-digest foods like soups and pureed dishes ensures that the body can absorb nutrients efficiently without additional stress on the digestive system.

Months 4–6: Immune- and Energy-Boosting Meals

Breakfast: Greek yogurt with berries and granola, smoothies with spinach and banana.

Lunch: Grilled chicken or fish with mixed greens salad, whole grain pita with hummus and veggies.

Dinner: Slow-cooked stews with lean beef or chicken, quinoa, and steamed broccoli.

Snacks: Energy bars, trail mix with nuts, and dried fruits.

These months emphasize foods high in antioxidants, omega-3 fatty acids, and probiotics to boost the immune system. Energy-boosting snacks help maintain stamina and vitality throughout the day.

Months 7-9: Anti-Inflammatory and Hydrating Meals

Breakfast: Avocado toast with scrambled eggs, whole grain waffles with fresh berries.

Lunch: Grilled chicken or fish with brown rice and steamed asparagus, lentil soup with whole grain bread.

Dinner: Roasted vegetables with lean beef or turkey, quinoa, and green beans.

Snacks: Fresh fruits, carrot sticks with hummus, dark chocolate.

Anti-inflammatory foods like turmeric and ginger help reduce inflammation, which is crucial during recovery. Hydrating foods ensure that the body remains well-hydrated, aiding in overall health and recovery.

Months 10–12: Recovery Meals and Mindful Eating

Breakfast: Omelets with vegetables and whole wheat toast, whole grain cereal with almond milk.

Lunch: Grilled chicken or fish with mixed greens salad, whole grain pita with hummus and veggies.

Dinner: Slow-cooked stews with lean beef or chicken, quinoa, and steamed broccoli.

Snacks: Energy bars, trail mix with nuts, and dried fruits.

These months focus on high-protein foods, complex carbohydrates, and healthy fats to support the body's recovery. Emphasizing mindful eating practices ensures that food is enjoyed and digested properly, enhancing the healing process.

Additional Guidelines for a Graceful Plate

• ***Practice mindful eating:*** Eat slowly, savor your food, and practice gratitude for the nourishment it provides.

• ***Include a diverse range of colorful fruits and vegetables in your diet.*** *They are rich in essential vitamins, minerals, and antioxidants.*

• ***Choose whole grains over processed grains***. Whole grains offer more nutrients and fiber.

• ***Include lean protein sources and healthy fats.*** These support muscle repair and overall health.

• ***Limit added sugars, salt, and saturated fats.*** These can lead to various health issues.

• ***Stay hydrated:*** Drink plenty of water and electrolyte-rich beverages.

Embracing the Graceful Plate for Liver Cancer Recovery

For liver cancer patients, nutrition plays a critical role in supporting treatment and recovery. The following sample meals are designed to provide liver-friendly nutrition over the course of a year.

Months 1–3: Balanced and Nourishing Meals

Breakfast: Oatmeal with fruit and nuts, scrambled eggs with whole wheat toast.

Lunch: Grilled chicken or fish with quinoa and steamed vegetables, lentil soup with whole grain bread.

Dinner: Roasted vegetables with lean beef or turkey, brown rice, and green beans.

Snacks: Fresh fruits, nuts, and carrot sticks with hummus.

These meals focus on providing balanced nutrition, with an emphasis on lean proteins, whole grains, and a variety of vegetables.

Months 4–6: Immune-Supporting and Energy-Boosting Meals

Breakfast: Greek yogurt with berries and granola, smoothies with spinach and banana.

Lunch: Grilled chicken or fish with mixed greens salad, whole grain pita with hummus and veggies.

Dinner: Slow-cooked stews with lean beef or chicken, quinoa, and steamed broccoli.

Snacks: Energy bars, trail mix with nuts, and dried fruits.

These meals incorporate foods rich in antioxidants and omega-3 fatty acids to support the immune system and provide sustained energy.

Month 7-9: Anti-Inflammatory and Hydrating Meals

Breakfast: Avocado toast with scrambled eggs, whole-grain waffles with fresh berries.

Lunch: Grilled chicken or fish with brown rice and steamed asparagus, lentil soup with whole grain bread.

Dinner: Roasted vegetables with lean beef or turkey, quinoa, and green beans.

Snacks: Fresh fruits, carrot sticks with hummus, dark chocolate.

Anti-inflammatory foods help reduce inflammation, while hydrating foods ensure the body stays well-hydrated.

Months 10–12: Recovery and Mindful Eating

Breakfast: Omelets with vegetables and whole wheat toast; whole grain cereal with almond milk.

Lunch: Grilled chicken or fish with mixed greens salad; whole grain pita with hummus and veggies.

Dinner: Slow-cooked stews with lean beef or chicken, quinoa, and steamed broccoli.

Snacks: Energy bars, trail mix with nuts, and dried fruits.

These meals focus on high-protein foods, complex carbohydrates, and healthy fats to support recovery. Mindful eating practices enhance the enjoyment and digestion of food.

Liver-Friendly Foods

Leafy greens: spinach, kale, and collard greens are packed with vitamins and minerals.

Cruciferous vegetables: broccoli, cauliflower, and Brussels sprouts promote liver health.

Berries: blueberries, raspberries, and strawberries are abundant in antioxidants.

Fatty fish: Salmon, tuna, and sardines provide essential omega-3 fatty acids.

Nuts and seeds: Walnuts, almonds, and chia seeds offer healthy fats and protein.

Healthy fats: Olive oil and avocado provide monounsaturated fats that support heart and liver health.

Embracing the Grace Plate means committing to a lifestyle of balanced, nutrient-dense eating that supports your body's natural healing processes. By choosing wholesome, nutritious foods and practicing mindful eating, you can enhance your overall health, boost your immune system, and improve your quality of life.

Remember, your body is your most valuable asset. Treat it with the love and respect it deserves by nourishing it with the Grace Plate. This approach to eating will not only support your recovery but also promote long-term health and vitality.

As you continue on your journey towards better health, let the Grace Plate be your guide. Make thoughtful food choices, practice mindful eating, and celebrate the positive impact that good nutrition has on your life. *Here's to a future of health, happiness, and grace—one mindful bite at a time.*

Chapter 9: Bridging the Nutritional Gap with Supplements

In today's fast-paced world, meeting our daily nutritional requirements through diet alone has become increasingly challenging. Modern agriculture, food processing, and lifestyle choices have all contributed to a decline in the nutritional value of our food. As a result, many people struggle to obtain the essential vitamins, minerals, and other nutrients necessary for optimal health. This chapter explores the reasons behind this nutritional gap and the role of supplements in bridging it.

As much as we strive to maintain a balanced diet, the reality is that obtaining all necessary nutrients solely from food can be challenging. Our modern lifestyles often lead us to make food choices based on convenience rather than nutritional density. Additionally, factors such as soil depletion, food processing, and cooking methods can diminish the nutrient content of our foods. Over the past century, significant changes in agriculture and food production have led to a noticeable decline in the nutritional content of our food.

The nutrient content of food can vary widely based on factors like farming practices, soil quality, storage conditions, and cooking methods. For instance, fresh produce may lose nutrients during transportation and storage.

Intensive farming techniques have led to soil depletion, where the soil lacks essential minerals and nutrients that would otherwise be transferred to the plants we eat. This can result in produce with lower nutrient content than in the past.

Many food processing techniques, such as canning and refining, can strip foods of essential vitamins and minerals. Cooking methods like boiling can leach nutrients into the cooking water, reducing their availability in the food itself.

Furthermore, factors such as age, gender, health conditions, and lifestyle choices (like smoking or alcohol consumption) can increase the body's demand for certain nutrients, making it harder to obtain adequate amounts solely through diet.

Given these challenges, nutritional supplements can play a vital role in filling the gaps in our diet. Supplements offer a convenient way to ensure you're getting essential nutrients, especially when dietary intake is insufficient or when specific nutrients are lacking in your diet. Supplements can provide a concentrated source of essential nutrients, ensuring that the body receives what it needs to function optimally.

Supplements are designed to provide concentrated doses of specific vitamins, minerals, or other nutrients that may be lacking in your diet due to dietary restrictions, preferences, or inadequate intake. Unlike food, where nutrient content can vary, supplements provide a consistent and measurable amount of nutrients, allowing for precise control over your intake. Supplements can be tailored to meet individual needs, such as during pregnancy, for athletes, or for individuals with specific health conditions that require higher nutrient levels.

While supplements offer a practical solution to nutritional gaps, it's important to make informed choices. When considering supplements, it is essential to choose high-quality products and consult with healthcare professionals to ensure they meet your specific needs.

Look for supplements that are tested for quality and purity by third-party organizations. This guarantees that the product contains the ingredients stated on the label and is free from any contaminants. Choose supplements with forms of nutrients that are easily absorbed and utilized by the body. For instance, methylcobalamin is a more bioavailable form of vitamin B12 than cyanocobalamin.

Ensure that the supplement provides an appropriate dosage based on your individual needs. Too much of certain nutrients can be harmful, so it is crucial to follow recommended guidelines and consult with a healthcare professional. Check the ingredient list for any fillers, additives, or allergens that you may want to avoid. Opt for supplements with minimally unnecessary ingredients. The role of regular check-ups cannot be overemphasized. Regular check-ups with your healthcare provider can help monitor your nutritional status and identify any deficiencies. Blood tests and other assessments can also guide your supplement choices and ensure you are meeting your needs.

But most importantly, supplements should complement, not replace, a balanced diet rich in whole foods. They are meant to enhance nutritional intake, not serve as a substitute for healthy eating. For instance, vitamin D is crucial for bone health, immune function, and inflammation regulation. It's produced by the skin when exposed to sunlight. Yet, many people lack sufficient sun exposure, particularly in winter. Vitamin D supplements can assist in maintaining adequate levels.

Omega-3 fatty acids found in fatty fish, flaxseeds, and walnuts are crucial for heart health, brain function, and reducing inflammation. Many people do not consume enough omega-3-rich foods, making supplements like fish oil or algae oil beneficial.

Magnesium plays a role in more than 300 biochemical reactions in the body. It supports muscle and nerve function, helps regulate blood sugar, and promotes bone health. Magnesium-rich foods include leafy greens, nuts, and seeds, but many people do not get enough from their diet.

Iron is essential for oxygen transport and energy production; iron is particularly important for women of childbearing age, who are at higher risk of deficiency. Iron supplements can help prevent anemia and support overall energy levels. B vitamins, including B12, B6, and folic acid, are essential for energy production, brain function, and DNA synthesis. Vegetarians and older adults are at higher risk of B12 deficiency and may benefit from supplementation. Calcium Crucial for bone health and muscle function, calcium is found in dairy products, leafy greens, and fortified foods. Those who do not consume enough calcium-rich foods may need supplements to maintain bone density and prevent osteoporosis.

In conclusion, while striving for a balanced diet remains crucial, the reality of modern lifestyles and dietary habits often necessitates additional support, and supplements offer a practical and effective solution to bridge the nutritional gap by providing essential nutrients that may be lacking in our daily food intake. By understanding the challenges of obtaining all required nutrients from food alone and leveraging the benefits of high-quality supplements, you can empower yourself to achieve optimal nutrition and overall well-being. Integrating supplements into a balanced diet and healthy lifestyle can help ensure we meet our daily nutritional requirements and thrive in the face of modern challenges.

Remember, the goal is not perfection but a balanced approach that supports your health and vitality. By incorporating supplements wisely into your routine, you can ensure you're meeting your body's nutritional needs more effectively. The key is finding a graceful, balanced approach that supports your health.

Chapter 10: Embracing the Journey - A Summary and Action Plan

As we come to the end of this book, it's time to reflect on the journey we've taken together through the concept of GRACE and how it can transform our lives. Each chapter has provided insights, personal stories, and practical advice to help you navigate the complexities of life with grace. Now, we'll summarize the key points from each chapter and present a realizable action plan to help you integrate these principles into your daily life.

As we conclude this journey through the concept of grace, let's take a moment to reflect on the key lessons we've learned and how they can be applied to our lives.

Grace as a Guiding Principle: Grace is a powerful guiding principle that can transform our lives. By embracing grace, we cultivate kindness, compassion, and resilience, allowing us to navigate life's challenges with strength and positivity.

Setting Intentions and Goals: Setting clear intentions and goals gives us direction and purpose. It helps us stay focused and motivated, enabling us to achieve our aspirations.

Resilience and Adaptability: Developing resilience and adaptability allows us to bounce back from setbacks and embrace change. It empowers us to face challenges with confidence and determination.

Acceptance and Letting Go: Acceptance and letting go are essential for finding peace and contentment. By focusing on what we can control and releasing what we cannot, we create space for growth and happiness.

Nurturing Relationships: Healthy relationships are vital for our well-being. By fostering open communication, spending quality time, and expressing gratitude, we build strong, supportive connections.

Balance and Moderation: Balance is key to a harmonious life. Avoiding extremes and striving for moderation in all aspects of life helps us maintain well-being and avoid burnout.

Living Authentically: Embracing our unique path and staying true to our desires allows us to live authentically. It empowers us to make decisions aligned with our values and passions.

Healthy Nutrition: Nutrition plays a crucial role in our overall well-being. By choosing nutrient-dense foods, practicing mindful eating, and respecting our bodies, we support our health and vitality.

Realizable Action Plan

To help you integrate these principles into your daily life, here is a realizable action plan:

1. Daily Reflection: Spend a few minutes each day reflecting on your goals and intentions. Write down any insights or adjustments needed.

2. Practice Kindness: Perform one act of kindness each day, whether it's a compliment, a helping hand, or a simple smile.

3. Build Resilience: Identify one challenge you're currently facing and brainstorm potential solutions. Take a little step towards overcoming it.

4. Embrace Acceptance: Practice mindfulness meditation for 5–10 minutes each day to cultivate acceptance and presence.

5. Strengthen Relationships: Reach out to a loved one each week for a meaningful conversation. Express your gratitude and appreciation.

6. Find Balance: Evaluate your weekly schedule and make adjustments to ensure a balance between work, rest, and play.

7. Live Authentically: Set aside time each month for self-reflection and goal-setting. Ensure your actions align with your values and passions.

8. Eat Mindfully: Plan your meals ahead of time, focusing on nutrient-dense foods. Practice mindful eating by removing distractions during meals.

9. Stay Hydrated: Consume adequate amount of water throughout the day. Aim for at least 8 glasses to maintain hydration and promote overall health.

10. Celebrate Progress: Do this by acknowledging your achievements, regardless of their size. Use them as motivation to continue progressing.

As you embark on this journey of embracing grace and integrating these principles into your life, remember that change takes time and effort. Be patient with yourself and recognize that every small step you take brings you closer to a healthier, happier, and more fulfilling life. By setting intentions, practicing kindness, building resilience, and nurturing relationships, you create a foundation for a life filled with grace.

Embrace your unique path, live authentically, and treat your body with the respect it deserves. With the Grace Plate as your guide, nourish your body and soul, and watch as you transform into the best version of yourself.

Thank you for joining me on this journey. May you continue to live with grace, embracing each moment with kindness, resilience and gratitude.

About the Author

Chris S. Moses is a globally renowned author, trainer and expert in strategies to prevent child custody interference, international child abduction, and domestic violence. With a wealth of experience in epidemiology, child and maternal health and project management, Chris has trained and consulted with organizations worldwide sharing his expertise in victim assistance services, diversity inclusion and bias/unconscious bias.

As a seasoned author and trainer, Chris has written extensively on topics such as child and elder abuse, compassion fatigue, criminal justice and domestic violence. His work has been widely acclaimed for its insight and expertise. He has successfully passed a thesis on domestic violence/victim assistance with distinction and has recommendations for publication.

Chris's impressive background includes leading an anti-corruption organization in the Benin Republic, advocating for social justice and democracy and working as a Human Rights Activist and Journalist. He has also honed his writing skills as a bilingual Literary Editor at Edmonds Community College.

Through his work, Chris offers a unique blend of academic, professional, and personal expertise making him a sought-after authority in his field. As the CEO/Founder of PIPC Consulting LLC, Chris continues to inspire and empower individuals and organizations worldwide.

www.ingramcontent.com/pod-product-compliance
Lightning Source LLC
Chambersburg PA
CBHW051307250726
48656CB00004B/1531